Melody of Blooms

Redefining Pregnancy in Today's India

Rogini Sudarshan

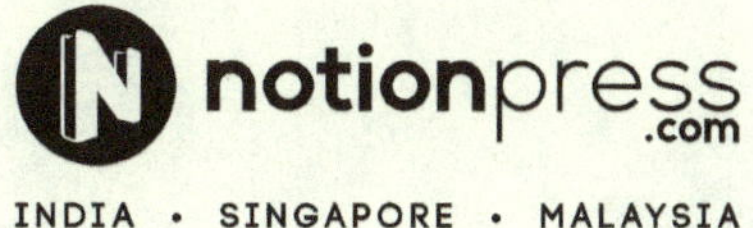
notionpress.com

INDIA • SINGAPORE • MALAYSIA

ISBN 979-8-89066-949-0

Table of Contents

Introduction

In the cacophony of a crowded Indian bazaar, amid the aroma of spices that permeate the air and the colors of life that swirl like a vivid tapestry, lies the quintessence of the nation itself: diversity. India, a land of myriad tongues, faiths, and customs, is also a country that reveres the essence of creation—motherhood. It is here that I, your humble guide, step onto the streets to take you on an odyssey through the labyrinthine tales of pregnancy in modern India.

Picture this: a young woman draped in a vibrant saree, her hands adorned with colorful glass bangles, her forehead graced by the sacred bindi, and her baby bump covered by her saree to ward off the evil eye. She is the embodiment of tradition—a soon-to-be mother cradled by centuries-old customs. As she walks, her smartphone pings—a reminder for her prenatal yoga class. In this vivid imagery, two realms entwine—the ancient and the contemporary. These strings weave together the chorus that resounds throughout this book—stories of hope, trepidation, and love.

But before we delve into the book, let us pause for a moment and ask ourselves a question: What does it mean to be pregnant in today's India?

Through a tapestry of voices from the grassroots to the metropolitan, this book seeks to unravel the enigma that cloaks pregnancy and answer this question.

India has always held motherhood on a divine pedestal. From the veneration of goddesses epitomizing fertility to rituals such as "*Godh Bharai*" and "*Seemantham*" that celebrate the expectant mother, pregnancy is sacralized. This divinization, however, is fraught with contradictions. Beneath this reverent façade lie several currents that flow against the tide. One such current is the preference for male offspring, which is deeply rooted in the Indian culture and has often led to abysmal practices such as gender-based abortions.

But change is in the air, like the gentle zephyr that heralds a new dawn. Contemporary India is witnessing a generation of women and men who are breaking these shackles. Women, buoyed by education and economic independence, are reshaping the contours of their pregnancy experiences. They are asserting their agency in the choices surrounding their pregnancy—right from the decision to become a mother to the modes of childbirth.

India's diversity casts varying shades on this narrative. On the one hand, urban landscapes depict women as multitaskers who juggle career, homemaking, and parenthood. On the other, rustic landscapes tell tales of women for whom motherhood is less of a choice and more of a compulsion.

A 2016 study conducted by the Indian Journal of Community Medicine indicates that over 50% of pregnant women in India, particularly in rural areas, do not receive adequate antenatal care. This is in sharp contrast with urban centers, where tech-savvy mothers-to-be use mobile apps to track their pregnancy milestones.

Take a dive into the past, and you will encounter a plethora of myths surrounding pregnancy—some enchanting, others bewildering. Tales abound of how cravings were believed to be whispers from the unborn, how an eclipse could curse the child in the womb, and how the expectant mother's thoughts could mold the baby's destiny.

Modern times have not quite escaped the clutches of mythology. Today's myths wear new attire—from consuming saffron to have a fair-skinned child to avoiding the consumption of shellfish to prevent birthmarks. These contemporary myths, endorsed through social media and word of mouth, shape the narrative of modern Indian pregnancy.

Let us now turn our attention to fathers. In contemporary India, fathers are breaking the stereotypes. They are now active participants, right from prenatal classes to the delivery room. A study by MenCare, a global fatherhood campaign, found that Indian fathers' participation in daily tasks related to parenting has increased significantly over the past few years.

This book is an invitation to witness this metamorphosis of pregnancy in India. It's an endeavor to dispel the taboos, herald the triumphs, and hold a flashlight to the challenges that lie ahead.

As you turn the pages, let the stories they tell resonate with you. Let the confluence of traditional and modern practices take you on an unforgettable journey through the very heart of India—raw, resilient, and resplendent.

First Trimester

The Paws and Claws of Pregnancy: A Guide to Safe Pet Ownership

Me and my husband, Ram, share a deep love for animals. Our home is filled with the delightful presence of three adorable cats, whom we consider our furry children. They have brought immense joy and warmth to our lives. When I discovered that I was pregnant, it was a moment of both surprise and gratitude for us. Little did we know at the time that this journey would require us to make some changes in our routine pet-handling methods to ensure the safety and well-being of our growing family.

As any responsible pet owner would know, the risk of toxoplasmosis during pregnancy is a grave concern. Toxoplasmosis is an infection caused by a parasite that can be found in cat feces. While our cats are loving companions who are vaccinated and well-cared for, my doctor advised us to take extra precautions with our pets to minimize any potential risk to the child. This was not an easy task, as our cats were accustomed to snuggling with us, seeking our affection, and being part of our daily routines.

To create a safe environment for our growing baby, we had to make some changes that felt like a temporary separation. We introduced a separate bed for the cats in another room, altering their routine of sleeping alongside us. We did this to ensure that they had their own space and to minimize my potential exposure to any infections that they might carry. It was a challenging adjustment, as I longed to snuggle with my furry children; but I knew that this adjustment was essential for the well-being of our baby.

Throughout my pregnancy, I often felt torn between my affection for our cats and the need to prioritize the health of our unborn child. It was as if I had to temporarily set aside the role of being a cat parent to ensure the well-being of our little one. It was a bittersweet sacrifice, but one that I knew was necessary.

The arrival of our baby girl brought us immense joy and relief. It was heartwarming to witness the incredible bond that developed between our cats and our precious bundle of joy. Our cats seemed to understand that our baby girl was a part of our family, and they instantly became her protectors and constant companions. Seeing them cuddle together and share tender moments filled my heart with gratitude and reassurance.

Now, as I reflect on this journey, I am overwhelmed with happiness. Our cats have seamlessly embraced their new role as guardians and playmates to our baby girl. Their gentle demeanor and unwavering love create an environment of comfort and security for our little one. Witnessing their interactions with our baby fills me with a profound sense of fulfillment and gratitude.

Although being a pet parent during pregnancy required certain adjustments and sacrifices, the rewards have been immeasurable. Our home is now filled with the harmonious presence of our beautiful daughter and our beloved furry children. It is a testament to the power of love and the unique bonds that can form between humans and animals. I feel incredibly blessed to have such a loving and caring family, both human and feline, to share this incredible journey of parenthood.

When it comes to handling pets and pregnancy, there are certain precautions that need to be considered; but it is entirely possible to have a safe and fulfilling experience. One concern that is often raised is the risk of toxoplasmosis, which is an infection caused by the parasite Toxoplasma gondii. While cats are commonly associated with this infection, it is important to understand how it is transmitted.

Toxoplasmosis can be contracted through the ingestion of contaminated or undercooked meat, or by coming into contact with infected soil or vegetables. Cats, particularly outdoor cats, may become carriers of the parasite when they consume infected birds or rodents. It is, therefore, crucial for pregnant pet mothers to practice good hygiene habits to minimize the risk of disease transmission. This includes refraining from cleaning the litter box yourself, avoiding contact with stray cats, washing hands thoroughly after interacting with cats or soil, and ensuring that vegetables are thoroughly washed and meat is properly cooked.

As a responsible pet owner, it is also important to ensure regular health check-ups and vaccinations for your pet. Keeping them healthy and up-to-date on vaccinations is not only beneficial for their well-being but also helps reduce potential risks during your pregnancy.

Preparing your pet for the arrival of a baby is another crucial aspect to consider. If you have a cat or dog, it is essential to familiarize them with the sounds and cries of a baby to avoid any adverse reactions when the baby actually comes around. Changing their routines gradually can also help them adjust to the new dynamics of the household. Introducing some flexibility in waking times and meal schedules can help make the transition smoother, considering the demands of caring for a newborn.

Furthermore, it is vital to continue giving attention to and spending quality time with your pets even after the baby arrives. Neglecting your pets due to the demands of the baby can lead to feelings of loneliness and depression in your furry companions. Including them in activities involving the baby and ensuring that they feel valued and loved can help prevent the arising of any negative emotions or jealousy.

While the bond between pets and their owners is special, it is crucial to establish boundaries for the safety of both your baby and your pet. Avoid allowing pets to sleep or sit in the baby's bed, as this can pose potential risks to the baby. Pets may become overly excited or seek warmth and comfort, thereby increasing the chances of accidents. Taking steps to secure your baby's sleeping area can help prevent any undesirable incidents.

Having pets during pregnancy can offer numerous benefits, such as emotional support and opportunities for physical activity, especially if you have a dog that requires regular walks. Additionally, growing up with pets can have positive effects on children, such as fostering empathy, responsibility, and companionship in them.

While precautions are necessary, it is entirely possible to enjoy the companionship of pets during pregnancy. By taking the appropriate measures, practicing good hygiene, and ensuring the well-being of both your pet and your baby, you can create a harmonious and joyful environment for everyone involved.

The Fitness Pulse: Embracing Exercise During Pregnancy

I have always found solace and joy in the world of sports and fitness. Zumba, yoga, and cycling were my passions long before I discovered the precious gift of life growing within me. I crave the exhilaration of movement, the rush of endorphins, and the sense of harmony between mind and body that I achieve while engaging in these activities. When I learned about my pregnancy, these passions did not waver, but rather grew stronger.

Fortunately, my pregnancy was smooth and healthy, and my doctor saw no reason for me to stop doing what I loved. However, the harmony in my life was disrupted by the concerns put forth by my family. I knew they meant well, but felt disheartened by their words of advice, which were filled with caution and worry. Every Zumba move, every cycling trip, and every yoga pose was met with warnings of potential harm to my baby and the fear of a miscarriage.

As a mother-to-be, I found myself in a delicate balancing act. On one hand, I wanted to prioritize my health and continue with my sports and fitness routine. On the other hand, I wanted to respect the concerns of my loved ones. It was challenging to navigate through their misunderstandings and criticisms. But deep within me, I had unwavering confidence in my body and its ability to protect and nurture my unborn child, even during moments of physical activity.

Every criticism and doubtful look hurt. The warnings lingered in my mind long after they were spoken. Yet, I held onto my conviction that I was making the right choices. While I understood the love and fear that fueled their concerns, I also knew that my body was capable and strong. I was doing what felt best for both myself and my baby.

I tried to bridge the gap of understanding through countless conversations, explanations, and sharing of the advice given by my doctor. However, changing deeply ingrained beliefs proved to be an uphill battle. In their eyes, my growing belly was a symbol of vulnerability that demanded constant protection and caution, not the exhaustion from practicing Zumba or yoga.

But those moments of activity were the only times when I felt most alive, liberated, and healthy. To have those experiences tainted by unfounded worries was disheartening. Still, I remained steadfast in my resolve, knowing that I was contributing to a healthier and happier pregnancy journey for both me and my baby.

Exercise during pregnancy is a much-debated topic. While some shroud it in layers of taboo, modern medicine and research vouch for its myriad benefits, quoting that pregnancy is in fact uncomplicated and healthy. Engaging in moderate sports or exercise during pregnancy is not just safe but beneficial.

If you were active during your pre-pregnancy period, maintaining the same level of activity is generally safe and encouraged. Regular exercise during pregnancy can improve your posture, uplift your mood, reduce discomfort, and even decrease the risk of gestational diabetes. Most importantly, it can equip you with the strength, endurance, and confidence required during labor and delivery.

Starting a new strenuous activity during pregnancy, especially without prior experience, is not advisable. However, initiating a mild exercise regime under the guidance of your doctor can be beneficial. A simple routine like walking is considered safe and beneficial.

The American College of Obstetrics and Gynecology recommends 30 minutes or more of moderate exercise per day for pregnant women. But not all exercises are for everyone. Some could be uncomfortable or harmful for pregnant women.

Some general guidelines to follow include avoiding exercise in hot conditions and high altitudes, being cautious not to lose balance while exercising, and steering clear of contact sports in which there is a risk of impact.

Despite taking these precautions, if any discomfort or abnormal signs appear, it is paramount to consult your doctor immediately. Pregnancy is a journey of joy; it should never be made at the cost of safety. With the right knowledge, guidance, and precautions, embracing fitness during pregnancy can add a vibrant rhythm to this beautiful journey.

Rainbow Pregnancy: A Journey of Healing and Hope

The day I found out that I was pregnant again, a mix of emotions raced through my heart. I felt as if someone had whipped up happiness, gratitude, and a tinge of sadness and poured it all over me. Although memories of my past loss still lingered in my mind, I felt hopeful and ready to start this new phase of my life. At 28, working in IT and running a busy life in the bustling city of Chennai, I knew that I was about to embark on a journey that would change me forever.

I couldn't forget the pain of my previous miscarriage. It was like a faint scar that I could always feel even if it was not visible. That bitter experience had made me more cautious. Every move I made and every decision I took felt like it needed an extra layer of thought. I was doing my best to protect and nurture the tiny life inside me.

As days turned into weeks, I was on a tightrope, trying to balance the happiness and the worries. Chennai, with all its noise and love, felt like it was waiting with bated breath, just like me. Simple things like a cup of coffee in the morning felt special, and I was always on high alert for any sign of something going wrong.

My first ultrasound had an oddly calming effect on me—it was almost like time had slowed down. Seeing that little heartbeat on the screen was pure magic. It reminded me that life, however small, is precious and awe-inspiring.

Of course, I still had those moments when my heart would sink. Hearing unfortunate stories or thinking about what could go wrong would sometimes overshadow my happiness. But then, I'd gather myself and say, "This is different, and I'm doing everything I can to keep my baby safe."

Here's the thing—my heart was carrying a story—a story that started with tears but was turning into a beautiful journey. I learned that there is a term for this experience—"rainbow pregnancy"—a symbol of hope and healing. Although the pain of my past miscarriage could not be erased from my mind, this new chapter was teaching me how strong and hopeful we can be.

Standing at the starting point of this journey, my heart mixed with the happy present and the stormy past, I decided to give it my all. The little movements in my belly were the sweetest reminders of the life growing inside me, and my nights were filled with dreams and whispered hopes.

The whispers of a tiny voice, the miniature heartbeat that promises a new beginning, and the dreams woven around it can sometimes be rudely snatched away by the untimely end of a pregnancy. Miscarriage, which is an often unspoken grief, can leave a deep void in the hearts of expectant parents. When life takes such an abrupt turn, the path to becoming pregnant again is laden with fears, uncertainties, and shadows of the past.

Statistics reveal that about 10 to 20 percent of known pregnancies conclude in miscarriage, often before the 12th week. This data, however, only skims the surface as countless miscarriages occur so early that the pregnancy might have not even been known.

This commonality though, does not diminish the heartache a miscarriage brings. The tapestry of emotions is complex and fraught with anxiety for women who tread the path of pregnancy post-miscarriage. To them, every flutter and every doctor's visit might seem like a roller coaster ride.

It is vital to recognize that these emotions are natural. As American author and grief counselor Dr. Earl A. Grollman said, "Grief is not a disorder, a disease, or a sign of weakness. It is an emotional, physical, and spiritual necessity, the price you pay for love. The only cure for grief is to grieve."

In such delicate moments, a cocoon of support, empathy, and understanding becomes essential. Both partners need a sanctuary to grieve, accept, and rebuild the fragments of their dreams. Professional help, compassionate counseling, and sometimes just an understanding ear can pave the way for emotional healing.

In recent years, a term describing this very situation has gained prominence—"Rainbow Baby." This is a term that is used to refer to a child born or adopted into a family that has previously experienced a miscarriage, stillbirth, or neonatal death. The metaphor of a rainbow symbolizes hope and light following a storm or a period of darkness and turbulence. It is a poignant depiction of joy emerging from a place of profound sorrow.

While the birth or expectation of a rainbow baby can be a time of immense joy, it can also bring about a flurry of complex emotions. Rainbow pregnancies can sometimes assist the parents to heal from the previous loss, and provide a glimmer of hope in an otherwise harrowing experience. Yet, they can also be marked by heightened anxiety, guilt, and even fear.

A significant aspect of navigating this complex emotional landscape is the recognition and acceptance of these feelings. It is crucial to understand that feelings of fear or constant monitoring of the fetus's growth and development are natural reactions to past traumatic experiences.

What's equally important is the process of acknowledging the baby who was lost. For many parents, naming the lost baby and assigning them a place within their family serves as a vital part of their healing journey. It keeps the memory of the lost baby alive, while also creating space for a new life.

Open lines of communication within the family is essential during this period. Honest and heartfelt conversations can provide much-needed support and understanding for the expecting mother. Additionally, regular mental health check-ups for both parents-to-be are of paramount importance.

Navigating pregnancy after a loss is no small feat. It is a journey that requires strength, resilience, and a tremendous amount of support. But amid all the anxiety and fear, there lies the hope for a rainbow after the storm, a testament to the unwavering strength of the human spirit.

Remember, it's okay to feel joy, it's okay to feel fear, and it's okay to miss the baby you lost while anticipating the one you're about to meet. You're not alone in this journey, and every step you take will take you closer to your rainbow.

As societies, we must foster an environment where grief can be openly expressed, where support is extended without judgment, and where couples are empowered to embark on their pregnancy journey with renewed hope and vigor after experiencing a miscarriage.

A majority of women go on to have successful, healthy pregnancies following a miscarriage. This resilience, coupled with support and understanding, can serve as the building blocks of a new journey.

Exploring Pregnancy's Heightened Sense of Smell

As I embarked on the journey of pregnancy with my husband Rishi, in the bustling city of Bangalore, our lives took on a new rhythm. We had always been meticulous in our work and shared a passion for keeping our home pristine. Rishi used to tease me about my obsession with cleanliness; but there was something comforting about the scent of a fresh and spotless house.

Expanding our family was a decision that we made with careful planning. We attended prenatal classes and immersed ourselves in learning about the ins and outs of pregnancy. We knew there would be discomforts and changes in our bodies, like nausea and fatigue, but what I experienced went beyond what I was prepared for.

One of my senses suddenly became supercharged—my sense of smell. It was like the world around me had transformed into a symphony of fragrances, each one distinct and vivid.

Every scent became more intense, more alive. The sweet aroma of jasmine flowers sold by the local vendor would fill our home with a beautiful fragrance, like a poetic melody. The tempting smell of my neighbor's *sambar*, which is a mouthwatering South Indian dish, would waft into our house, igniting my appetite.

But this heightened sense of smell also came with certain challenges. It made me highly reactive to less pleasant odors as well. The overpowering perfume worn by a stranger sitting next to me on a bus could be extremely unsettling. During my first trimester, when morning sickness clung to me like a parasite, even the slightest unpleasant smell could send me running to the nearest restroom.

The intensity of my sense of smell was disorienting, at times even overwhelming. But it became another part of my intricate journey of pregnancy. Slowly, I learned to adapt and manage. I always carried mints and scented lotions to counter any unwelcome odors. I became more mindful of my food choices, avoiding triggers that could worsen my persistent nausea.

Amid it all, I discovered that pregnancy is a multi-sensory experience. It awakened me to the subtle nuances of the world around me. Each scent had its own story and its own memory, and became a part of the intimate experience that I began sharing with my growing child.

Around two-thirds of pregnant women find themselves presented with a heightened sense of smell, particularly during their first trimester. This peculiar development, often termed "hyperosmia," can make the ordinary scents of daily life seem incredibly vivid. Researchers have connected this amplified sense of smell to the fluctuating hormone levels in pregnancy, and believe that it may sometimes contribute to morning sickness.

In India, which is a country that is rich in diverse scents, this might mean that expectant mothers would experience the smells around them in a profoundly intense way. India's tapestry of aromas, from the earthy scent of monsoon rains to the tempting fragrance of street food, can become an even more striking experience.

But it's not all rosy; the potent smells can also become overwhelming. Therefore, it would be wise for expectant mothers to find ways to manage this newfound sensitivity. Simple measures like ensuring good ventilation at home, offloading some cooking duties to avoid strong kitchen smells, and maybe keeping a pleasant-scented sachet nearby can be surprisingly effective.

Pregnancy is a journey in which the expectant mother's body is adapting and evolving to support new life. It is like a dance in which sometimes the music is soft and tender, and sometimes it swells to a dramatic crescendo. It is important for pregnant women to recognize and understand these changes, and maybe even embrace them as part of the incredible journey of bringing a new life into the world.

As Benjamin Franklin once said, "Change is the only constant in life. One's ability to adapt to those changes will determine your success in life." Embracing and adapting to the changes during pregnancy, even the amplified scents, is part of the beautiful path to motherhood.

Timing the Big Reveal: Deciding When to Share Your Pregnancy News

As a 27-year-old working professional living in Chennai, my life has followed a carefully plotted path thus far. But then, an unexpected twist appeared on my horizon—I discovered that I was pregnant. Mixed emotions flooded my being. While a part of me was overjoyed, another part was worried about the impact of this change on my career aspirations. A promotion was within reach at the time, and the pregnancy felt both thrilling and daunting.

Navigating the professional world as a pregnant woman can be complex. The weight of managing the expectations of impending motherhood alongside my career ambitions bore down on me. So, my husband Kumar and I decided to keep our little secret to ourselves for the first three months. Those early weeks felt like a delicate balancing act, cherishing the secrecy while grappling with the physical changes taking place within me.

Managing the familiar symptoms of pregnancy, like morning sickness and frequent trips to the restroom, while striving to maintain my professional façade, was no small feat. Fatigue became my constant companion, often leaving me breathless as I tackled my daily work responsibilities. I became a master of crafting creative explanations to deflect any suspicions about my condition.

One particular morning stands out in my memory. Overwhelmed by nausea, I sought solace in the restroom, splashing cold water on my face. Just as I was trying to compose myself, a colleague walked in, and her eyes filled with curiosity on seeing me. In that tense moment, I quickly attributed my discomfort to some disagreeable food, and she nodded sympathetically. I breathed a sigh of relief, knowing my secret was safe... at least for now.

As the weeks progressed, maintaining the delicate balance between work and pregnancy became increasingly challenging. Fatigue clung to me like a shadow, making it harder to divert my thoughts from the miracle unfolding within me.

Sharing the news of a pregnancy is a special moment that couples get to decide on. Many couples choose to wait until they hit the three-month mark. This isn't just a random number. Doctors usually advise waiting until the first trimester is over, as this period is critical for the baby's development.

During the first three months, the little one builds its base in the womb. Everything from the heart to the brain starts to form. This is an extremely delicate stage. During this time, there is a high chance of things not going as planned. Statistics say that between 10 and 20 percent of known pregnancies end during the first three months.

For working women, announcing their pregnancy at work can be kind of a roller coaster ride. There is the joy of sharing the news, but also the worry about how the boss and colleagues might react.

A study conducted by Penn State University in 2018 says that women who get positive reactions at work when they shared their pregnancy news tend to have a happier pregnancy. That's how much a supportive work environment matters.

In the end, when to share the news is a personal decision. Some like an early celebration, while others prefer to wait for the right moment. Ultimately, it's your news and your story. Pick the time that makes you feel confident and happy. Be it early or a little later, it's all about sharing the joy.

Second Trimester

Ties that Bind: Exploring Parenthood Together

When I, Anitha, discovered that I was carrying a new life within me, a rush of emotions engulfed my heart. Excitement and apprehension danced together, mingling with countless questions and concerns. How would motherhood reshape me? Would I rise to the challenge of nurturing another human being?

My marriage to Deepak, arranged in the traditional style, had brought a delightful mystery into my life. Hailing from a modest town in Tamil Nadu, I was a fiercely independent woman working in the bustling city of Chennai. So, taking a break from my career to have my baby seemed inconceivable. But as my pregnancy progressed, the idea of cherishing every milestone of my baby's life started to shift my perspective.

Yet, I couldn't help but wonder how this impending arrival would affect Deepak, my companion on this uncharted journey. Would he embrace fatherhood with the same fervor as he did his work?

Weeks turned into months, and I witnessed an astonishing transformation in Deepak. A newfound energy seemed to fuel his every move. He became more invested and more devoted in ensuring that everything was just right. It left me intrigued, wondering what had sparked this sudden change.

Deepak and I had been unraveling the depths of our relationship since our marriage two years ago. However, the thoughts and fears about my impending motherhood, along with the idea of pausing my career, were sacred to me. I hesitated to burden him with these concerns, unsure of how he would react.

One serene evening, while driving home from a routine doctor's appointment, Deepak broke the silence. With a calm voice and a determined gaze, he unveiled his wish: He was striving harder than ever so that I could enjoy the privilege of staying home with our baby. His words, unexpected as they were, struck a deep chord within me.

As an independent woman who took pride in her career, the idea of becoming a stay-at-home mom felt foreign. But as I absorbed Deepak's earnestness and his aspirations for our future, I started to see the beauty in his proposal. The opportunity to witness our baby's every smile, every word, and every tentative step became an enticing prospect, a privilege too precious to overlook.

This revelation deepened my love for Deepak. I admired his unwavering commitment to our family's well-being and his willingness to make sacrifices. It opened my eyes to a new perspective, where the joy of motherhood and the bonds of family outweighed any professional ambitions.

The path to parenthood had begun, and I knew it would be an awakening, shaping us in ways we couldn't yet fathom.

Anitha and Deepak's stirring story is a window into the transformative journey that pregnancy brings for both men and women. In the Indian society, where family values run deep, the expectant father often takes on the mantle of a provider with renewed vigor. This, as we saw in Deepak's case, is a common reaction. But let's take a closer look.

While the expectant mother delicately cradles the life blossoming within her, the father's connection with the unborn child takes a unique form. Men, who may not experience the same physical and emotional journey as women do during pregnancy, often have their own ways of expressing joy and excitement. Some become more serious, driven to ensure financial security for their family, like Deepak. Others become more caring, taking on household responsibilities and being present for their partner. For some men, the realization of impending fatherhood dawns upon them only when they witness the growing baby bump.

Interestingly, some fathers-to-be exhibit symptoms mirroring those of their pregnant partners, a phenomenon known as "Couvade syndrome" or sympathetic pregnancy. Weight gain, constipation, nausea, fatigue, and even mood swings can manifest in these men; some may even experience pain during labor! While the exact cause of this reaction is yet to be fully understood, theories suggest that empathy for their partner and hormonal changes contribute to this temporary condition. Couvade syndrome becomes a rite of passage for men on their journey to parenthood.

In the realm of pregnancy, mothers and fathers have their own unique experiences, and it is important for both of them to acknowledge and understand these individual paths of each other as they embark on the remarkable journey of parenthood.

As American author and speaker, Pam Leo, beautifully put it, "Let's raise children who won't have to recover from their childhoods." This sentiment resonates with many fathers-to-be, like Deepak, who intensify their efforts to lay a strong foundation for their growing family.

Recent studies have supported this observation. A survey conducted in 2019 by the National Family Health Mission in India revealed that 68% of men accompanied their spouses on their prenatal care visits. This reflects the changing dynamics and the evolving involvement of Indian men in the journey of pregnancy.

But, it's crucial to understand that the load of expectations should not weigh too heavily on either parent. The shared joy of ushering a new life into the world should be coupled with shared responsibilities and open communication. This openness creates a haven for both the mother and the father to foster not just the growing life, but also the relationships that bind the family.

In a society in which people's roles are constantly changing, it is the weaving together of support, love, and understanding that creates the fabric of a nurturing environment for a child to be born into. Through shared experiences and emotions, couples like Anitha and Deepak are painting a new picture of parenthood for the generations to come.

The Long-Awaited Bloom: The Joys and Fears of a Long-Awaited Pregnancy

Here I am, Revathi, a 32-year-old woman, finding solace in the loving embrace of our home in Pune. My husband, Mani, has been my constant companion on this journey, and together, we have walked hand-in-hand for seven years. Every month, our hearts would flutter with hope, yearning for the day our dreams of starting a family would come true. But time passed, and our hopes wilted, leaving us in the shadows of unfulfilled longing.

After much turmoil, Mani and I decided to take a leap of faith into the world of IVF. The road ahead was steep and financial constraints loomed over us, but we were quite hopeful. We became frequent visitors of the fertility clinic, which was filled with stories of hope and heartbreak. We embarked on our first attempt, wishing for a delicate bud and a promise of new beginnings. But as luck would have it, the fetus didn't take root, leaving us devastated.

Our doctor's gentle words reminded us that miracles sometimes need more than one chance. Though our resolve was shaken, it remained unbroken. So, we tried a second time.

Then, like a ray of sunshine breaking through the clouds, our miracle happened: We were finally going to have a baby of our own. Our families shared our elation, but their excitement came with a touch of overprotectiveness. Their advice, meant to ensure my safety, started to confine me, overshadowing the joy of my pregnancy. They cautioned me against engaging in several activities, including everyday actions like climbing the stairs, and urged me to take complete bed rest. While I understood their concerns, I felt trapped and unable to fully enjoy my journey.

I knew the importance of taking care of myself and the baby, but I also knew my own body and what I was capable of. With the guidance of my doctor, I was able to find a balance between engaging in various activities and ensuring the safety of my baby. I embraced gentle activity and modified my routine to prioritize my well-being and the health of our baby. I wasn't being reckless; I was only trying to reclaim my autonomy and cherish this precious time.

Throughout this challenging period, Mani stood by my side, as a pillar of support. His understanding and unwavering belief in me gave me the strength to navigate the maze of advice and worries. Our doctor too, provided invaluable guidance, helping me find the confidence to live my life while keeping our baby's well-being in mind.

When a couple has been trying to have a baby for ages, and then—boom!—pregnancy happens, it's like hitting a jackpot. The moment is filled with so many emotions for the couple and their families. You can almost hear the fireworks!

But here's the thing: This amazing news sometimes comes with a side of worries. The family might turn into an overprotective squad, and the mom-to-be might become stressed about making sure that everything goes perfectly. Now, it's good to be cautious, especially if this is a rainbow pregnancy—that's when a pregnancy happens after miscarriages or failed fertility treatments. But being too cautious and turning the mom-to-be into a bubble-wrapped package? Not so much.

It is essential to know that not every pregnancy needs extreme measures like total bed rest or stopping all daily activities. We're all unique, and so is every pregnancy.

Now, don't get me wrong—making some lifestyle changes and taking precautions is wise. But it's all about finding that sweet spot where the mom-to-be can still enjoy her pregnancy journey. This is where a trusty doctor comes into play. Doctors are like the wise owls of pregnancies. Follow their advice to strike the right balance.

One more thing—communication is key. Talking to family members openly and calmly about the pregnancy can help in keeping things smooth. And if there is someone who is extra worried (you know, the kind who wants to wrap you in bubble wrap), here's a tip: Take them along to a prenatal appointment. Let them see the baby through an ultrasound or hear the heartbeat. Trust me—it's a game changer! They will see that everything is going well, and it can be a magical moment for them too. They might then loosen their grip on you.

Remember, a pregnancy after a long wait is like a rare gem. Handle it with care, but don't forget to let it shine!

Ask, Discover, Embrace: Empowering Questions to Ask During Pregnancy

In the exhilarating world of pregnancy, my practical mind desired clarity. I, Praveena, a 30-year-old founder of a marketing company, thrive on knowing the ins and outs of everything that comes my way. My pregnancy, as expected as it was, opened a new page in my life's narrative, and I couldn't wait to pen down each and every detail. I took the reins early, and at six months, I was well into my prenatal classes, and labor preparations were on my radar.

Doctor's visits felt like my research hours, and each one was a chapter I was eager to dive into. I'd walk in, my mind abuzz with questions—you could say my thoughts were as organized as my work presentations. It was important to me that my medical team and I were in sync; their expertise was the anchor to my ship in these uncharted waters.

However, what I envisioned as a collaborative quest sometimes felt rushed, leaving me grappling for the reassurance I sought. Despite this, my resolve stood unshaken; I knew the importance of understanding my journey and ensuring that my voice was heard.

Each appointment, sadly, was reminiscent of a fleeting shadow, a mere five-minute blur where my meticulously prepared list of queries was met with cold efficiency rather than empathetic understanding. The hurried nods of my doctor, the perpetual chime of the door indicating the next patient entering the clinic, the teeming waiting room—everything was nerve-racking. My concerns and my anxieties seemed to evaporate into thin air before they could be meaningfully addressed, leaving me grappling with more doubts than before. It was disheartening to witness the doctor's demeanor change as I ventured to ask more questions, as though I was disrupting the assembly line of her daily routine.

I did not wish to be just another name on the doctor's appointment list, just another tick mark on her checklist. I yearned for empathy, understanding, and patient guidance, not hurried consultations and unsatisfactory responses.

The relentless pressure and intimidation, however, did not deter me. If anything, it served as a catalyst, fortifying my resolve to advocate for myself and my child. I firmly believed that my health and my baby's well-being were not matters to be rushed or neglected. And while it was crucial to respect the physician's time, it was equally important to ensure that my concerns were addressed satisfactorily.

My predicament, I soon realized, was not an isolated experience. Many women, especially first-time mothers navigating the tumultuous seas of pregnancy, share similar tales. Intimidation and apprehension often muzzle our voices, preventing us from asking critical questions and expressing our concerns.

In the journey of pregnancy, finding the right doctor and hospital is like finding the right travel guide and stay for an important trip. These choices can make a huge difference in how the journey feels and how the memories are made.

Many people, especially first-time expectant parents, often feel shy or nervous to ask questions when they visit the doctor. This is common.

However, it's crucial to remember that this is your journey, and the doctor is there to guide you.

A study that was published in the Journal of Pregnancy and Child Health in 2019 reported that patients who actively engaged with their healthcare providers by asking questions and discussing concerns had more positive experiences during their pregnancy and childbirth. It's just like having a tour guide—if you don't ask questions, you might miss out on some fantastic destinations!

Now, let's talk about the importance of comfort level with your doctor. The pregnancy journey is intimate, and so, your relationship with your doctor should be based on trust. In Indian culture, family members might pressurize the parents-to-be to go to a specific doctor or hospital; but it's important to listen to your own instincts too. If you don't feel a connection or comfort, it's absolutely okay to switch. Take it like trying out a different hotel if the first one doesn't meet your needs.

Bear in mind that having your medical records handy is like having your travel documents in order—it makes transitions smoother. If at any point, something feels off, or you just need a bit more assurance, getting a second opinion is akin to checking reviews for that hotel you're not so sure about.

Remember, pregnancy is one of life's most profound journeys, and having the right companions and settings can help in turning it into a cherished memory. Trust yourself, engage actively, and don't hesitate to make the choices that feel right for you.

Wisdom and Boundaries: Finding Your Path Through Pregnancy Advice

In the lively town of Erode, the news of my pregnancy filled the air with excitement. As a 29-year-old teacher working at a local play school, I felt embraced by the warmth of my community. My husband and I had just celebrated our first year of marriage, and the arrival of our baby added an extra sparkle to our lives.

Being unable to visit my parents owing to my husband's busy work schedule, I found solace in the loving embrace of my in-laws. Their care and support made me feel cherished and protected throughout my pregnancy journey.

Suddenly, I was the town's trending topic. I was drowning in a sea of advice about the dos and don'ts of pregnancy. An uncanny sense of disembodiment took over me and I felt as if I was on the sidelines, observing the control of my own body shift from my hands to the hands of the world.

Every imaginable opinion relating to my pregnancy, from my dietary habits to the expected weight gain, from birth preparation to infant care, was thrust upon me. As a first-time mother-to-be, I felt besieged by the barrage of contradicting suggestions. To top it all, it wasn't just my immediate circle who had adopted the role of advisory board; even strangers took the liberty to halt me mid-walk, inquire about my trimester, and smother me with their well-intentioned yet intrusive wisdom. There were those who, without any provocation or consent, thought it appropriate to touch my belly as though it were a communal treasure on display.

While it was endearing to witness their enthusiasm, it also became overwhelming. Everywhere I went, people would share advice about what I should or should not do. It felt like I was constantly under scrutiny, as if my body and my choices were no longer solely my own.

Initially, I tried to embrace the attention and take it in stride. But as months passed, the constant stream of advice became exhausting. I longed for a sense of autonomy and to make decisions based on my own instincts.

Looking back, I understand that the townsfolk meant well and their actions came from a place of love. However, it taught me the importance of setting boundaries and reclaiming ownership of my pregnancy journey. I learned to smile politely, nod, and filter the advice that came my way.

Through this experience, I realized the significance of trusting myself, seeking guidance from healthcare professionals, and prioritizing my well-being and that of my baby above societal expectations.

In the vibrant tapestry of Indian culture, where tradition and familial bonds thread through the fabric of society, pregnancy transcends a personal experience; it unfurls as a communal symphony. From the instant word of a pregnancy is whispered into the world, the expectant mother finds herself encircled by an ocean of advice and ancestral wisdom, not only from family and friends but also from the most casual of acquaintances.

There's a charm in this involvement, a testament to the closely woven nature of Indian communities. A myriad of advice cascades from every direction, mostly born from genuine care and concern. However, for good or for worse, pregnant women in this setting often metamorphose into public property—closely watched and incessantly commented upon during pregnancy and even after the child is born. The deluge of advice can be of various forms—some helpful, some bewilderingly amusing, others uncomfortable, and yet some that can scratch at the soul and flood an expectant mother's senses.

This swirling maelstrom is particularly formidable for first-time mothers who feel borne down by the weight of societal expectations, which may joust against their own instincts or the counsel of healthcare professionals.

Navigating these swirling currents necessitates both education and the adept art of boundary-setting. Prenatal classes serve as lighthouses, guiding expectant mothers with fact-based knowledge on pregnancy and childcare. Equally crucial is the skill of drawing a gentle, yet firm line around oneself. The sea of advice cannot be dammed, but it can be navigated.

Here are a few pointers to hold onto:

Stay calm and let your smile be your shield. *Oftentimes, a smile coupled with silence is a response that requires no further explanation.*

Master the art of deflection. *A subtle change in conversation can help you steer away from unsolicited advice.*

Keep responses succinct. *When engaged, opt for brief affirmation or polite negation —a simple "yes" or "no".*

Establish your own perimeters. *Discern what you'll embrace and what you'll gently let pass by. Remember, if someone is disconcerted by your choices, that burden is not yours to shoulder.*

Sometimes, **a polite but direct word** *can cordon off the unending stream of advice. Do this with a smile, so as to not ruffle any feathers.*

Embrace the truth *that it's your body, your pregnancy, and your baby. The choices you make and the paths you choose are inherently yours.*

There is an old saying that perfectly fits this scenario: "Take the advice that works for you, and politely nod for the rest." When the day wanes and the stars take their watch, this journey is intimately yours. It's woven into your very being. Being informed and steadfast in your choices is the compass by which you must navigate.

The Intimate Waves: Embracing Changes in Libido During Pregnancy

In our cozy apartment, David and I embarked on our married life, as a journey of adventure and exploration. Our marriage, which was an arranged union that felt like fate, was built on shared passions and a zest for life's simple pleasures. We were always open to new experiences and embraced the joys of companionship.

When pregnancy ventured into our lives, it brought along a whirlwind of changes. The first trimester was filled with nausea and exhaustion, but as I entered the second trimester, an unexpected change occurred. It was as if a gentle breeze had swept away the weariness, leaving me with renewed energy and a radiant glow.

What surprised me was that this newfound vitality went beyond physical energy. It awakened my senses and deepened our connection as a couple. I felt alluring and desired, igniting a flame of closeness between us. It was like an adventure within an adventure, another layer of our journey as we eagerly awaited the arrival of our little one.

However, this change brought its own set of challenges. My husband, though attracted to me, expressed concerns about the safety of our baby during our intimate moments. His worries cast a shadow over our physical connection, causing a strain that we hadn't anticipated.

At first, I felt rejected and hurt by his hesitation. I longed for the intimacy that we had shared before my pregnancy and felt that my newfound empowerment was being stifled. But I also understood his concerns and the need for a compromise. Together, we sought answers and guidance, turning to online resources and prenatal classes to address our shared anxieties.

Gradually, my husband's apprehension diminished, and was replaced by understanding and acceptance. He cautiously broached the subject, and we embarked on the journey of rediscovering our physical intimacy during this transformative time. We proceeded with care, ensuring mutual comfort and respect.

The result was an incredible experience that reaffirmed our bond and brought back the joy of intimacy into our lives. It became a testament to the power of communication, understanding, and empathy in navigating the challenges of pregnancy.

Looking back, this period of our lives was a profound learning experience. It tested us, but ultimately strengthened our relationship. The ultimate reward was the birth of our healthy, beautiful baby, as a testament to the love and resilience that we had cultivated together.

Let's talk about the core of the experience of David and Banu; this is something that's not always in the spotlight—changes in libido during pregnancy. Now, for a lot of women, this can be like a seesaw. Sometimes the mood is way up, sometimes it's way down. It's all natural.

Here's what happens. During pregnancy, the body gets busy with a hormone party. Estrogen and progesterone are like the VIPs at this party. When their levels go up, more blood flows to places like the genitals.

For some women, this means their libido might get stronger, especially in the second trimester.

Why the second trimester? Because it's like a sweet spot in pregnancy. The early symptoms like morning sickness and tiredness often fade away during these months. So, some women feel more energetic and might experience an increase in libido.

But that's not the story for everyone. For some, the sex drive might take a dip. The growing belly, changes in the body image, or even worries about the baby can affect how a woman feels sexually.

The American College of Obstetricians and Gynecologists says that changes in libido during pregnancy are normal. They suggest talking openly and honestly with your partner about how you feel.

Also, it's good to have a chat with your doctor. They can tell you if it is safe to have sex during your pregnancy and answer any questions that you may have.

Remember, there is no one-size-fits-all when it comes to how you feel sexually during pregnancy. It's like riding a wave—everyone's ride is unique. It's about what feels right and safe for you. So, communicate, be informed, and embrace the changes.

The Lullaby of Connection: Fostering Bonds in the Womb

The air was electrified with anticipation as Deepak and I sat hand in hand, waiting for the doctor to give us the news we were yearning to hear. The moment we learned that I was pregnant, it felt like time had frozen. The room was brimming with joy, laughter, and happy tears. We were going to embark on the most magical journey of our lives.

Five months rolled by like a whirlwind. Our tiny bundle of joy was growing inside me, and I was in awe of the miracle of life. Deepak was my steadfast pillar of support. He was there at every turn—ultrasounds, prenatal classes, and doctor's appointments. He'd read every book he could find on parenting and would often share little nuggets of information that he found fascinating.

Our last visit to the doctor was particularly memorable. She mentioned that our baby could hear us now. Talking, singing, or even humming to the baby could foster a beautiful bond. This revelation sent Deepak over the moon. He took up a mission to ensure that our child would recognize his voice from day one.

But here's where our paths diverged. Deepak found such joy in speaking to our baby; his voice was always filled with love and excitement. He would narrate stories, sing lullabies, and sometimes just ramble about his day.

For me, however, it was a different story. I felt this odd barrier that kept me from talking out loud to the baby. It felt like speaking into an abyss, and the silence that echoed back felt haunting. I was plagued with questions. Why couldn't I do what seemed so natural to Deepak? Was something wrong with me? Did I lack the motherly instinct that should have kicked in by now?

Days turned into weeks, and my inability to communicate out loud with my unborn child began to wear me down. I felt inadequate and torn. I loved my baby with every fiber of my being; but why couldn't I express it like Deepak did? I found myself feeling isolated, even though I was surrounded by love.

One quiet evening, as I sat by the window, I had an epiphany. There is no said way to express love. It is as diverse as the people who feel it. Deepak was expressing his love through words and songs, but maybe I was expressing it in some other way.

I realized that I too had been communicating with my baby, although not through words. My hands caressing my belly, the gentle massages, even the silent tears of joy—these were my love letters. My heart sang lullabies even if my lips didn't.

I decided to embrace my way of bonding with my baby and stopped measuring my love through spoken words alone. Deepak, ever the supportive partner, stood by me. We knew our little one was enveloped in the symphony of our love—his songs and my silent serenades.

As we prepared for the arrival of our bundle of joy, we knew that they would be welcomed into a world where love knows no bounds or barriers.

In the tapestry of pregnancy, an intricate thread of bonding weaves its way through, linking the mother and the child in an ethereal dance. This bonding often unfurls silently, without any conscious effort. The mother's heartbeats become the lullabies that cradle the unborn child, and the gentle rhythm of her breath becomes the child's calming mantra.

As the weeks roll by, the womb becomes a sanctuary where the bond between the mother and the child deepens. The soft pressure of the mother's hand massaging her belly, the whisper of lullabies, the vibrations from a speaker playing classical music placed near the belly, and the silent utterance of a name chosen with love—these are the threads that weave an unbreakable bond.

Meditation and reading books aloud also foster a serene environment for the baby. These moments of tranquility resonate through the mother's body, enveloping the child in warmth and security. The conversations that a mother has with her unborn child are akin to sowing seeds of love and trust that will bloom throughout their lives together.

By the time the baby is 18 weeks old, they begin to discern the sounds within the mother's body—the cadence of her heartbeat, the rumble of her stomach, and so on. As the child reaches the sixth or seventh month, they start listening to the whispers of the world outside the womb. The mother's voice becomes a known comfort, and the surrounding sounds lay the groundwork for their burgeoning awareness.

Studies have illuminated the immense benefits of communicating with the baby during pregnancy. When the soothing tones of a mother's voice wash over the baby, it instills a sense of calm and security. This communication is not just sound—it is the bedrock upon which the child's emotional and social development is built. It also plays a pivotal role in language acquisition and memory enhancement.

However, not all mothers find it easy to talk out loud to their unborn child. This does not make their love any less profound. For those who struggle with communicating with their baby, visualizing the child cradled in their arms while immersed in soothing music can sometimes bridge the gap. The emotions that cascade through them as they communicate in silence, reach the child through the placenta, caressing the little one with every heartbeat.

Traditional practices often incorporate elements that foster this bond. For example, in a tradition called "valaikappu," bangles worn by the mother are believed to create soothing sounds that resonate with the baby whenever the mother's hands are near her belly. These sounds are like echoes of affection that envelop the child.

Ultimately, it is important for the mother to engage in activities that bring her joy and contentment, as these emotions release hormones that bathe the child in happiness. The symphony of love that is created in the sanctuary of the womb is composed of many notes, each as vital as the other, crafting a melody that will resonate through the lives of both the mother and the child.

Redefining Roles: Navigating Pregnancy in a Nuclear Family

At 25 weeks pregnant, my life is undergoing a massive change. As a working woman in a nuclear family, I find myself caught in a balancing act. Each day brings new challenges—managing nausea while preparing for important work presentations, coping with fatigue and swollen feet while managing household chores, and navigating through unpredictable waves of emotions during high-pressure moments at work. It's a lot to handle, and often leaves me feeling emotionally drained and alone.

In the midst of it all, I long for emotional support. However, my partner, engrossed in his own work, feels distant. We seem to have less and less time for each other, and it leaves me feeling disconnected and lonely. There are moments when all I crave is a listening ear, a warm hug, and the comfort of having my partner share this incredible journey with me. But the demands of our daily lives often make it challenging to find those precious moments of connection.

Living in a nuclear family has its pros and cons. While it gives us freedom and space, we miss out on the collective wisdom, shared responsibilities, and a sense of belonging that come with extended family. As I navigate through the ups and downs of pregnancy, I find myself yearning for guidance from experienced elders or the companionship of siblings.

The roller coaster of hormonal changes, physical transformations, and psychological ups and downs leaves me feeling exhausted and isolated. Some days, the fatigue is overwhelming, and all I want to do is retreat to my bed and forget about the world. But responsibilities beckon, and I force myself to attend to the daily demands of cooking food, preparing for meetings, and taking care of household chores.

The transition from the realm of a joint family to the paradigm of a nuclear family is a growing phenomenon. While this shift comes with its fair share of advantages, it also amplifies challenges during significant life events like pregnancy. The absence of an extended support system during this period often precipitates feelings of loneliness and desolation.

In the shadows of such loneliness, the specter of prenatal depression can take hold. Prenatal depression, often overshadowed by its postpartum counterpart, is a mental health issue that is rarely discussed, although its impact is quite significant. According to the World Health Organization, approximately 10% of pregnant women worldwide experience depression during pregnancy. This condition, marked by persistent sadness and a loss of interest or pleasure in engaging in any activities, can have deleterious effects on both the mother and the child.

It is imperative that awareness around prenatal depression is amplified and that the silence surrounding it is shattered. Seeking help and opening up to someone during times of emotional turmoil is paramount. Through early intervention and support, pregnant women grappling with depression can find avenues to manage their mental health, safeguarding the well-being of both themselves and their unborn child.

Pregnancy is a physically exhausting and emotionally tumultuous period. The oscillating moods, fatigue, and hormonal surges can make even getting out of bed an uphill task. Therefore, having a helping hand can make a substantial difference.

Pregnancy marks the beginning of a journey of transitioning from being a couple to becoming parents. It is a period of transformation that requires space for redefining roles, responsibilities, and dynamics. Partners should proactively participate in the pregnancy journey of their spouse. Attending prenatal classes, accompanying for prenatal visits, and planning for childbirth together can have a profound impact on the pregnant mother's emotional health. A partner's understanding, emotional availability, and active involvement can serve as a beacon of support for the expectant mother.

Beyond the Norms: Navigating Pregnancy Without the Typical Symptoms

I am Rithika, a 31-year-old entrepreneur in Chennai. When I found out that I was expecting, a surge of emotions filled my being. I felt a mix of excitement and anticipation. My husband, Vicky, and I had been happily married for five years. All these years, we were entirely focused on our careers. Although we hadn't yet planned to start a family, life had different plans for us.

I had been around my sisters and sisters-in-law when they had their little ones, and supported them during their pregnancies. So, their experiences gave me an idea of what to expect, now that I was pregnant. I felt prepared, ready to face the ups and downs of this new journey.

But things took an unexpected turn. My pregnancy seemed smooth, without the usual morning sickness, cramps, and fatigue. This surprising calm left me worried. Was everything okay? Was this normal?

Vicky and I embarked on this new chapter with a mix of wonder and concern. The absence of familiar signs made me doubt if everything was progressing as it should.

I tried to embrace the tranquility and enjoy my relatively easy pregnancy. But over time, unease crept in. I longed for the expected signs, the reassurances that my body was nurturing new life. The absence of these familiar signs heightened my worries and created a chorus of anxieties.

The first trimester brought the most anxiety. Every trip to the bathroom became a moment of apprehension. The joy of pregnancy was overshadowed by constant worries. Each moment felt fragile, like I was walking on eggshells.

Only when my belly started to show did I allow myself some moments of joy. Yet, the fear of loss remained at the back of my mind, occasionally casting doubt on the journey.

The day of my first ultrasound gave me immense relief. Seeing the flicker of life on the screen brought happy tears to my eyes. It was just the confirmation that I needed.

Around the 25th week, I felt the first gentle movements of my baby. It was as if someone had blown tiny bubbles inside me, like the fluttering of butterfly wings. It was a magical moment, a reminder of the miracle growing inside me.

Looking back, I realize that my pregnancy was different. While many women experience common discomforts, mine was relatively calm. Each pregnancy is unique, and there is no right or wrong way to experience it.

Despite the uncertainties, I wouldn't trade my pregnancy for anything. It blessed me with a wonderful baby boy. His smiles bring me joy, and his laughter brightens my days. My journey through pregnancy taught me that even during life's quietest moments, extraordinary things can happen.

It's a fact that being pregnant doesn't always mean you'll have the usual symptoms. Each pregnancy and each woman is unique, and how each of us deal with pregnancy can vary. Many women experience the common symptoms, but not everyone. If you don't have the typical signs, it might make you anxious. In such cases, it's good to get your concerns addressed by your doctor; but it doesn't necessarily mean that something is wrong with your pregnancy or your baby.

Sometimes, a busy lifestyle can mask pregnancy symptoms. For example, a working woman might mistake pregnancy-related fatigue for just being tired from work. Mood swings might be brushed off as stress from work or personal life.

The bottom line is, you don't need to have all the usual pregnancy symptoms to be pregnant. Each woman's journey is different, and that's completely normal. Keep communication open with your doctor, and remember that a smooth-sailing pregnancy without the typical discomforts is not a bad thing. It's just a different, perhaps luckier, experience.

One Size Doesn't Fit All: The Truth About Diverse Baby Bumps

In the beautiful town of Karaikal, where the air carries a hint of salt and ancient traditions fill the atmosphere, I, Prabha, discovered the joy of pregnancy. At 26 years of age, with my loving partner Balu by my side, I embraced the blessings of starting a family.

As we shared the news with our families, a curious whisper spread through our close-knit community. You see, I have always been slender and active, thanks to my family's genes and my love for athletics. But as my pregnancy progressed, my baby bump remained a gentle curve, barely noticeable. This made our loved ones concerned. "Is everything okay?" "Isn't your belly too small for six months?" Their well-intentioned questions soon turned into a constant chorus, echoing in my ears.

I sought solace in my doctor's reassurances, but my family and friends remained convinced that I wasn't taking proper care of myself and the baby. Their concerns transformed into accusations, leaving me feeling overwhelmed and misunderstood. Every gathering became an opportunity for unsolicited advice, pressuring me to eat more and follow their ideas for an ideal pregnancy.

Despite my attempts to explain my doctor's evaluation and professional opinion, my words seemed to vanish into thin air. The pressure to conform to their expectations of a pregnant woman's appearance became relentless and draining. It felt as though I was on trial, my every decision being scrutinized.

In the midst of this chaos, I had an epiphany. This was my journey, my body, and my baby. I knew them better than anyone else. I made a conscious decision to trust my doctor's guidance and follow my instincts, disregarding the unsolicited advice and comments.

This wasn't an easy path, as the concerns and opinions persisted. However, I became stronger with each passing day, resilient in my determination to prioritize my well-being and my baby's health over baseless scares.

As my due date approached, my pregnancy progressed smoothly. My baby grew healthily, and my doctor affirmed our progress. This journey taught me the power of trusting myself and embracing the uniqueness of my pregnancy.

Reflecting on this transformative experience, I realized that it wasn't just about the physical changes or the development of a new life within me. It was a journey of self-growth, understanding my body, and asserting my decisions. I learned to block out external noise and trust my instincts, creating a space where I could celebrate the remarkable nature of my pregnancy.

Pregnancy is indeed an individual journey, influenced by many factors like genetics, lifestyle, and overall health. The shape and size of a baby bump are not accurate indicators of a baby's health or growth. Just like each baby is different, so is each pregnancy. Our bodies adapt in their unique ways to accommodate this beautiful process.

When expecting, particularly for the first time, it's common to have a neat baby bump due to tight abdominal muscles. However, as you move on to your second or third pregnancy, you might observe a more prominent bump since the stomach muscles may have loosened. Therefore, it is crucial to resist comparisons and unnecessary scrutiny. The focus should be on maintaining a healthy lifestyle and adhering to medical advice—that's the best we can do for our babies and ourselves. After all, a healthy baby comes in various sizes, as do healthy baby bumps.

As the above story shows, it is important to remember that only you and your doctor are in the best position to understand and decide what's best for you and your baby. While others may offer advice out of concern and love, always consider your doctor's advice and your understanding of your body as the ultimate guideline during your pregnancy.

The story also underscores the importance of advocacy. We must advocate for ourselves and our babies and trust in the beauty of our unique pregnancy journeys, no matter how divergent they may seem from popular perceptions or expectations. After all, there isn't a universal manual for pregnancy, and there isn't a "one size fits all" baby bump. It is as unique as the life it nurtures within.

Beyond the Pause Button: Balancing Career and Pregnancy

As pregnancy unfolded, my life took on a new meaning. As the Vice President of a successful company, my days were filled with purpose and challenges. My husband, Uthay, and I, two driven individuals, felt it was the right time to welcome a new life into our world.

Contrary to what some people believed, my work did not burden me. Our lives were a harmonious dance of responsibilities, where work and personal life intertwined seamlessly. So, we were able to cherish every aspect of our pregnancy journey.

But as my belly grew, so did the chorus of cautionary voices. Concerned individuals, a mix of traditionalists and well-meaning advisors, whispered about the stress and the need to slow down.

The truth is, my work wasn't a source of stress; in fact, it fueled me and gave me a sense of fulfillment. It was an integral part of me. Pregnancy wasn't a limitation; it was an expansion of my horizons. I was thriving in the corporate world, solving problems and meeting deadlines. Pregnancy didn't dampen my drive; it only added a new layer to my identity: a mother-to-be, determined to provide the best for my growing family.

Unfortunately, those around me expected my responsibilities to overwhelm me. They saw my ability to balance work and pregnancy as a ticking time bomb instead of a manageable feat. Unsolicited advice flowed in, tinged with worry and doubt. They urged me to take it easy, warning that I might harm the baby by continuing to work. Their concerns lingered in my mind, undermining my confidence.

But I knew in my heart that I could handle both my job and my pregnancy. The skepticism from others felt condescending and disheartening. My autonomy as a woman seemed to be disregarded. However, I refused to let their doubts cloud my conviction.

As time passed, the chorus of concern grew louder. People around me enquired about my health, not out of genuine care, but to assess if I was struggling. Every conversation seemed to be geared toward hearing me admit defeat.

In a world where women have proven their capabilities time and time again, it was disheartening to have to defend my choices repeatedly. I wasn't just balancing work and pregnancy; I was defending my capabilities and my right to make decisions for myself. It felt as if my entire identity was reduced to the bump on my belly.

But I refused to be defined solely by my pregnancy. I was a woman with a career I took pride in, actively shaping my future. I wouldn't allow guilt or societal expectations to dictate my choices.

So, I made a conscious decision. I listened to my body, consulted my doctor, and most importantly, trusted myself. I took the necessary breaks, prioritized self-care, and continued my work without compromising my health or the well-being of my child. I learned to filter out the noise of unsolicited advice and focused on my own well-being and professional growth.

Pregnancy is indeed a significant milestone, and each woman experiences it uniquely. It is not a Pause button on your life or career; it's another chapter. And this chapter, like all others, should be written by the woman living it. Pregnancy shouldn't box women into stereotypical roles. Women can manage numerous responsibilities. They can be both career-driven and nurturing mothers.

In a society that has successfully launched women into space, it is high time we understood that they can handle the pressures of career and motherhood simultaneously. It is imperative to acknowledge the strides women have made in various fields, including space exploration. Pregnancy doesn't incapacitate a woman; it only makes her stronger. And it's crucial that society supports and respects her choices.

Now, let's look at some practical advice for harmonizing career responsibilities and pregnancy. Staying hydrated is paramount, as is avoiding prolonged periods of sitting or standing. Regular intervals for short walks or gentle exercises are advisable. When it comes to attire, prioritize comfort. Moreover, it is wise to pace oneself and maintain a balanced diet. It is of utmost importance to be attuned to one's body and take adequate rest as needed. These strategies will contribute to a conducive environment for both professional success and a healthy pregnancy.

So, to all working expectant mothers—remember, your strength isn't defined by the doubts of others. Trust your capabilities, lean on your support system, and continue to chase your dreams. Remember, pregnancy doesn't pause your life; it merely enhances it.

And to everyone else—let's shift our mindset. Let's normalize women who choose to work during pregnancy and support them rather than doubting their ability. Let's change the narrative from how hard it's going to be for them to how we can support them. Because at the end of the day, it's her body, her pregnancy, and her choice.

Beneath the Surface: The Truths about Pregnancy and Gender

Throughout my pregnancy journey, which unfolded against the backdrop of a play school in Chennai, there was a unique and endearing aspect that colored our days. At 29 years, celebrating our first year of marriage, my husband and I were filled with joy when we discovered the whispers of new life awaiting to enter our home. The love and care from my in-laws embraced us, creating a warm and nurturing environment.

My father-in-law, with his radiant smile, would go out of his way to pick me up from work, providing support when my husband couldn't. And my mother-in-law, a talented cook, delighted in preparing meals that satisfied my every craving, enveloping me in her loving embrace.

Amid this loving tapestry, a playful tradition unfolded. My spirited mother-in-law became an eager investigator, determined to guess the gender of our baby. Like an explorer venturing into uncharted territories, she delved into age-old tales and folklore, searching for signs and symbols in my every move, sleep, and growing belly.

Initially, her gender-predicting adventures brought a sense of whimsy to our pregnancy journey, amusing us all. However, as time went on, her relentless guessing game became a repetitive tune, and I yearned for a break from her constant attention. Her unwavering focus felt suffocating, as if the weight of centuries-old mysteries rested on every breath I took.

While I was surrounded by love and care, the delicate fabric of my pregnancy became entwined with my mother-in-law's persistent guesses. The enchanting melody of impending motherhood danced alongside the tireless rhythm of her predictions.

Every craving I experienced, whether it was for tangy tamarind or sweet gulab jamuns, fueled her theories. "Ah, a taste for sweetness? It must be a girl," she would exclaim, her eyes sparkling with excitement. And when my belly sat high, she confidently declared, "Definitely a boy!"

Initially, I found her playful obsession endearing; a charming diversion from the usual conversations about morning sickness and mood swings. It was heartwarming to witness her anticipation and joy for the newest addition to our family.

However, as the weeks turned into months, her incessant speculation became a constant presence, like a repetitive drumbeat that never ceased. Every interaction seemed to revolve around her latest theory about the baby's gender. Although I knew it was all in good fun, the unrelenting scrutiny built up a sense of anticipation, keeping the actual revelation perpetually out of reach.

It is fascinating how deeply-rooted myths and age-old beliefs still persist in the modern world, especially when it comes to pregnancy. One of the common misconceptions that many people hold is the belief that the way a woman carries her baby or the cravings she experiences can help predict the gender of the child. These beliefs have been passed down through generations and, surprisingly, are still widely believed despite tremendous advancements in medical science.

In reality, the way a woman carries her baby is mainly influenced by her body type, muscle tone, and the position of the fetus—it has nothing to do with the baby's gender. Similarly, cravings during pregnancy are more likely linked to nutritional needs or hormonal changes rather than the gender of the baby. The American College of Obstetricians and Gynecologists affirms that there is no scientific evidence supporting the notion that the position or shape of the belly and cravings are reliable indicators of a baby's gender.

In the context of India, the desire to predict a baby's gender has more serious implications due to a history of gender bias. Unfortunately, some families in the past have shown a preference for male children, which has led to adverse consequences such as sex-selective abortions and skewed gender ratios. To counter this, the Government of India passed the Pre-Conception and Pre-natal Diagnostic Techniques (PCPNDT) Act in 1994, which makes it illegal to determine or disclose the sex of a fetus. This law is aimed at preventing sex-selective abortions and promoting gender equality.

Therefore, in India, the gender of the baby can be known only after the baby is born. The focus is rightly placed on the health and well-being of the mother and the child, regardless of gender.

While it can be entertaining to guess the baby's gender in family gatherings or baby showers through various old wives' tales, it is crucial to understand that these methods are not based on scientific facts. The beauty of pregnancy lies in the anticipation and the joy of welcoming a new life into the world, irrespective of its gender. Let's embrace this journey with openness and a commitment to love and nurture the child, regardless of whether it's a boy or a girl.

The Other Side of Pregnancy: Embracing the Journey's Ups and Downs

As I sit in my favorite armchair, raindrops dancing outside, I reflect on how my life has come full circle. As an entrepreneur in bustling Mumbai, my days are usually filled with appointments and the organized chaos of the city. But now, I find myself on the most unpredictable journey of all—motherhood. It all began with a simple plus sign on a pregnancy test, leading me through a tale of paradoxes and raw truths.

I feel compelled to share a feeling that may go against societal expectations. I have a confession to make about pregnancy, a phase that is often romanticized. Brace yourselves, dear readers, for I am about to be brutally honest. I did not enjoy being pregnant.

Yes, you read that correctly. The process of carrying my child brought profound discomfort and tested my endurance. My body, which was once my sanctuary, went through rapid and uncontrollable changes. I was a passenger, not the driver, on this journey. Cravings, mood swings, constant bathroom trips, and general unease were dictated by the tiny life growing inside me. Despite my efforts to surrender to these changes, I couldn't shake the feeling of losing control over my own existence.

Now, as a mother of a three-month-old baby, I am able to look back on that phase of my life with a bit more clarity. My feelings, though different from what society expects, were valid. They were my truth. However, I do understand that the challenges I faced during my pregnancy were the necessary steps leading to the joy and fulfillment that I now experience as a mother.

Breastfeeding my baby has been a transformative experience, deepening the bond that we share. It goes beyond the physical act, symbolizing our profound connection. It is a reminder of the incredible journey we have embarked on together.

Let's get real for a moment. Pregnancy is often painted as a time filled with sunshine and rainbows. Movies and TV shows make it look like a dream. But the truth? It's not always a bed of roses.

For some women, pregnancy can feel like a heavy weight. They might not enjoy the journey, and that's okay. It doesn't make them any less of a mother. Feeling this way doesn't mean that they don't love or won't love their baby. It's just that pregnancy itself might not be their cup of tea.

There's a whole platter of reasons for these feelings. Maybe it's the morning sickness that feels like an unwelcome guest. Or it could be the aching back and feet, or maybe feeling like a balloon ready to pop. For some, the reason could be deeper—maybe a past loss, or the pregnancy was unexpected. Sometimes, it's just a feeling of losing touch with oneself, as the body changes and hormones go on a roller coaster.

And guess what? They are not alone. A study by the University of Otago in New Zealand reports that many women face mixed emotions during pregnancy, including feeling down or anxious.

So, what can someone do if they're not enjoying pregnancy? Well, embracing the positive sides can help. Think about the little one growing inside. Some women find joy in doing maternity photoshoots or writing a pregnancy journal.

It's also important to have good pals around—people who would understand and support without judgment. And if the feelings get too heavy, talking to a healthcare provider or counselor would be a smart move.

In short, not enjoying pregnancy doesn't reflect negatively on anyone. It's a chapter in life, and like any other chapter, it has its ups and downs. What matters is that it's just one part of the amazing journey of bringing a new life into this world.

Third Trimester

Calling Fathers to the Frontlines of Pregnancy and Beyond

I'm Iniya, a resident of Chennai, blessed with a love story that unfolded amid the corridors of college and flourished in the office spaces where Selva and I worked together. As we embarked on our careers side by side, our relationship grew deep roots and enveloped our lives. Eventually, we tied the knot with the blessings of our families, sealing our commitment to each other.

And then, it happened. The thin pink line appeared on the pregnancy test, like an equator dividing the life we knew from the life that awaited us. That line completed the picture of our family, confirming our joyous news. We were going to have a baby. At that moment, our hearts overflowed with dreams and aspirations. We immersed ourselves in discussions about the future, imagining our child's features, laughter, and the milestones they would reach. Together, we were a team, ready to embrace the thrilling uncertainty of parenthood hand in hand. But little did we know about the silent isolation that lay ahead.

As weeks turned into months and my belly grew, a subtle shift began to unfold. My husband found himself being slowly pushed to the periphery. Our pregnancy check-ups, which were once shared experiences, became centered around me. The doctors and nurses directed their questions and discussions toward me, leaving my husband sitting quietly in the corner. Even during ultrasound sessions, which were the magical moments of seeing our baby, he often found himself sitting alone in the waiting room due to protocols. The joy that should have been shared became an increasingly solitary journey.

The same pattern emerged at home. Whenever my husband tried to express his feelings or actively participate in the pregnancy, he was sidelined. Dismissive comments, unsolicited advice, and the weight of societal expectations loomed over him. The prevailing narrative seemed to imply that he wasn't capable of understanding or navigating the journey of parenthood, diminishing his enthusiasm and excitement. It pained me to witness him being subtly and systematically pushed away from an experience we had envisioned as a shared journey.

This sense of isolation extended into the postpartum phase as well. With the arrival of our little bundle of joy, an unexpected wave of intrusion entered our lives. My husband, just as much a new parent as I was, found himself feeling out of place in his own home. His attempts to help or engage with the baby were often brushed aside by the "more experienced" elder women in our family taking over. His role in our child's life seemed reduced to that of a bystander.

The excitement, anticipation, fears, and anxieties of becoming a parent for the first time were just as real for him as they were for me. But where were his outlets? Who was there to acknowledge his silent struggles and provide support during his transformation?

One fine day, over a steamy cup of chai, my mum and grandmother started to reminisce the tales of yesteryears. My eyes widened as they casually spoke of how my own dad was practically a phantom presence when I was born. It's tradition, they murmured with a shrug—men were mere spectators while the women orchestrated the baby symphony.

Suddenly, a jigsaw piece clicked into place. Why had this lopsided arrangement become such an accepted norm? I looked at my husband, then at my adorable baby, and my heart clenched. Why should he miss out on the joy and bonding, the late nights and the first smiles?

That's when it dawned on me that this unspoken tradition was a relic of a deeply patriarchal past, where roles were rigidly defined. It was unfair and unjust, and I didn't want it casting a shadow over our little family's story.

There is a pressing need for a shift in the narrative of parenthood. Healthcare providers, families, and society as a whole need to recognize and validate the father's role in this journey. A concerted effort should be made to include them in prenatal appointments, childbirth classes, and postnatal care discussions. They too need support, reassurance, and a safe space to express their fears, doubts, and emotions.

Every child deserves an involved father, and every father deserves to be a part of his child's life from the very beginning. Let us encourage fathers to be a part of the prenatal and postnatal journey. Let's break down the barriers of stereotypes and biases that keep them in the sidelines. Let them be a part of the appointments, the ultrasounds, the breastfeeding classes, and the sleep training discussions. Let us understand that their concerns, fears, and anxieties are just as valid, and they too need to be heard. Let us create an environment in which fathers are not made to feel as if they are intruding into a feminine domain but are accepted as equal partners in parenthood.

And let us, as a society, educate ourselves to better understand and appreciate the role of fathers in pregnancy and postpartum care. Let's dispel the myths and misconceptions that shroud the concept of fatherhood. Let's celebrate not just motherhood but fatherhood too. The joy and satisfaction a father experiences from being a part of these crucial moments are invaluable and fosters a stronger bond between the father, the child, and the mother.

As we move toward a more inclusive society, it's essential to make fathers feel that they are an integral part of the pregnancy and postpartum journey. This is a call for a paradigm shift, to move away from exclusion and toward inclusion, creating a healthier, happier parenting experience. Because fatherhood, like motherhood, is not just a responsibility but a gift, an opportunity to love, nurture, and shape a new life. And that journey begins not when the child is born, but from the very moment they start growing in the womb.

So here's to more love, more inclusivity, and more understanding. Here's to fathers who stand by their partners during those prenatal appointments, to fathers who feel a lump in their throat at the first glimpse of their child in the ultrasound, and to fathers who aren't afraid to change diapers or handle a baby's midnight wailing. Here's to fathers everywhere who are striving to be a part of the beautiful journey of parenthood. You're not alone, and your role is just as important. The journey is challenging but the rewards are beyond measure.

In the end, parenthood isn't just about giving life; it's about participating in the act of love, nurturing, and raising a child together. It's a dance in which every step, every twirl, and every sway matters. And it takes two to tango.

Prenatal Classes in India: Breaking Misconceptions and Bridging Generation Gaps

As the countdown to the miracle of bringing a new life into this world ticked away, my heart swayed with a mix of excitement and apprehension. At 28 weeks pregnant, I embraced my new identity as an expectant mother. I sought knowledge through prenatal classes. It was like quenching my thirst for understanding, as I delved into the vast expanse of pregnancy.

In these classes, I discovered a sanctuary of understanding and connection. Stories and wisdom flowed, painting a vivid picture of the journey ahead. They instilled in me the clarity and confidence to navigate childbirth, not as a passive passenger, but as a captain steering my own ship.

But to my disappointment, my pursuit of knowledge was met with furrowed brows from the elder members of my family. They viewed my earnest quest as an indulgence, an unnecessary expense. In their eyes, childbirth was a river that had flowed through generations without the need for maps and compasses. They questioned why I felt the need to dive deep when the current would naturally carry me along.

Their unsolicited advice and criticism pierced through me, leaving me feeling unsupported and underappreciated. Their objections stemmed not from a place of disdain but from the confines of their experiences, which were devoid of such opportunities when they were in my shoes.

But my vision was unfettered. My journey into motherhood was not about the paved roads of the past, but the path I wished to carve for myself. Attending these classes was not merely about the physical act of birthing; it was a step toward gaining control over my experiences. It was about arming myself with information and empowerment, enabling me to make informed decisions that resonate with my beliefs and preferences for my baby and me.

The chasm between our perspectives was wide, fueled by generation gap and contrasting experiences. Despite their reluctance, I hoped they would understand the rationale behind my decisions and the value these classes held for me.

The skepticism I encountered was not surprising. The questions bombarded at me were familiar—Why attend classes when one could engage in household chores and remain active at home? I educated them that these classes were not merely meant to teach physical exercises but also incorporated theoretical aspects of pregnancy, labor, pain management, breastfeeding, and much more.

Prenatal classes, also known as pregnancy or childbirth classes, are an invaluable resource that is often overlooked. These classes serve the vital purpose of educating and preparing couples for the journey of childbirth, breastfeeding, postpartum care, and newborn care. While these classes have gained popularity in many parts of the world, in India, they are still a relatively new concept. This makes it challenging for new parents-to-be to convey their importance to older generations who may question their necessity.

One common misconception of our elders is that prenatal classes are solely focused on physical exercises. However, it is crucial to emphasize that these classes go beyond mere physical activity. They provide a comprehensive understanding of pregnancy, labor, pain management techniques, breastfeeding, and various other aspects of the journey to parenthood. In a time when information is readily available from numerous sources, it can be overwhelming to discern what is accurate and relevant. Prenatal classes offer reliable guidance, helping couples navigate through the abundant information and separating myths from facts.

It is important to bridge the generation gap and help our elders understand that times have changed. Lifestyles, work dynamics, our understanding of the human body, and even dietary patterns have evolved significantly. This understanding may take time to develop; however, it is essential to explain the purpose and content of these classes to our elders. In fact, involving them in the process by inviting them to attend the classes alongside you can be a powerful way to foster understanding and appreciation. Witnessing firsthand the wealth of knowledge and support offered in these classes may help dispel any doubts and foster a greater appreciation for their value.

As we embark on the journey of parenthood, it is crucial to seek knowledge and embrace new approaches that are based on scientific evidence and best practices. Prenatal classes provide a structured platform for learning, support, and empowerment. By promoting awareness and understanding among our elders, we can collectively recognize the significance of these classes in ensuring a healthy and fulfilling pregnancy journey for both the expectant parents and their loved ones.

Gestational Diabetes: The Uninvited Guest in Pregnancy

My husband, Krish, and I live in Coimbatore, which is a lively city full of colors and flavors. When we got to know about my pregnancy, we were quite excited about becoming parents. But a few months into my pregnancy, our excitement was dampened by a new development: I had gestational diabetes.

I got really worried. My doctor, though, told me that with changes in my diet and activity, the condition could be managed. I decided right then and there that I would do whatever it took to ensure the good health of my baby.

But, let me tell you, it was not a walk in the park. I am a foodie, and sticking to a strict diet was tough. And it wasn't just hard for me. We lived with our extended family, and meal times turned into a juggling act. My mother-in-law ended up cooking two separate meals—one for the family, and another just for me. She had to make sure that mine had less oil, no sugar, and avoid foods that would spike my blood sugar levels. White rice, idly, dosa—all were off the table for me. This meant extra work and attention in the kitchen.

As the months went by, my cravings went through the roof. I would have done anything for sweets, smoothies, biryani, and chaats. But I had to resist, and it made me so cranky and irritable. Going out became almost impossible because the temptations were everywhere. I ended up avoiding family functions and outings with Krish because I didn't want to face the food I couldn't have.

And then there were the comments from family and friends. Some meant well, but didn't understand my situation. "I ate everything when I had sugar during my pregnancy," one person told me. She didn't realize that her C-section was linked to her gestational diabetes. I was also told that I shouldn't exercise much and that I should rest more because I was pregnant. But in my heart, I knew what I wanted—a healthy pregnancy without medications or a C-section.

The guilt weighed heavily on me. I felt like I was burdening my family with the separate meals and felt guilty about my cravings and irritability. The struggle to keep up with the diet and exercise was both a physical and mental battle.

But you know what? I pushed through. I worked hard on myself for the sake of my baby. I want to say this to all expectant mothers facing similar challenges—it's essential to know your goals and stick to them. There's nothing wrong with setting boundaries and politely declining advice that doesn't align with what you know is best for you and your baby.

As my pregnancy drew to a close, I experienced the profound joy of welcoming a healthy baby girl through a natural birth. Holding my child, nourishing her, and witnessing the unbreakable bond of motherhood filled me with immeasurable gratitude and joy.

Gestational diabetes is like an uninvited guest that can sometimes show up during pregnancy. It's when blood sugar levels go up, usually around the second trimester. Why does this happen? Well, it's because of hormones from the placenta messing with how the body uses insulin, which is a hormone that helps the body in using sugar to generate energy. So instead of sugar going into the cells, it stays in the blood.

Now, here's a staggering fact: In India alone, a substantial number of women grapple with this condition annually, painting a sobering picture of its prevalence.

What's tricky is that gestational diabetes is like a ninja—it does not really show any symptoms. But there are some factors that make it more likely for a woman to get it—like being overweight, having had gestational diabetes in a past pregnancy, having polycystic ovary syndrome (PCOS), or having a family history of diabetes.

This sneaky nature of gestational diabetes often puts an extra burden on expectant mothers. Many women end up internalizing the guilt, thinking that their lifestyle choices might have led to the condition. It's a heavy weight to carry, especially when you're trying your best for the little one growing inside you. The struggle to maintain a diet when your body is screaming for the comfort of your favorite foods is real. Some days, it can feel like an uphill battle, especially when hormones are all over the place.

And here's why it's important to catch and manage gestational diabetes: It can create a domino effect of complications. It can lead to the baby growing too big, which makes C-sections more likely. It can cause the baby to be born too early, have low blood sugar after birth, or even have a higher chance of developing obesity or type 2 diabetes later in life. Moms aren't spared either—they also have a higher risk of developing type 2 diabetes down the road.

So, what can we do about it? Good news—it can be managed! Sometimes, eating healthy and staying active is enough. It's like giving the body the right tools to fight back. In other cases, medication might be needed to keep those blood sugar levels in check.

The bottom line is, it's super important for moms-to-be to work hand-in-hand with their doctor. Keep tabs on those blood sugar levels and follow a game plan that's best for both mom and baby. Consulting a nutritionist for a tailor-made diet can also be a great move.

It's crucial at this point for family and friends to rally around, offering support rather than judgment. Understanding, empathy, and encouragement go a long way in helping an expectant mother to stay positive and focused on her health and that of her baby. It's important to remember that while lifestyle can be a factor, sometimes these things just happen, and it's no one's fault. Together, with love and support, the journey can be made more bearable and even empowering.

Gestational diabetes might be an uninvited guest, but with the right steps, it doesn't have to take over the party.

The Complexities of HCG and Twin Pregnancies: A Deeper Look

My husband and I had been married for three wonderful years, cherishing our time together as a couple before venturing into parenthood. After much contemplation and heartfelt conversations, we finally felt ready to embark on the journey of becoming a family of three. With excitement and anticipation, we made the decision to stop using contraception and start planning for our long-awaited pregnancy. Little did we know that our plans would unfold quicker than we expected.

Just four months after discontinuing contraception, my period was late. So, I decided to take a home pregnancy test. The two pink lines that appeared confirmed our suspicions, and we scheduled an appointment with a doctor to validate the results. The doctor advised us to wait for the 40-day mark to conduct an HCG test, which is a crucial step in assessing the growth and development of the fetus. We anxiously waited, hoping for positive news.

The day arrived, and I underwent the HCG test. The results came back, and to our astonishment, the HCG levels were doubled. A mix of excitement and nervousness washed over us as the doctor performed an ultrasound to check the positioning of the fetus in the uterus. I couldn't help but notice a slight look of confusion on the doctor's face as she repeated the scan. My heart was beating fast, and a thousand thoughts raced through my mind. Finally, the doctor turned toward us, a smile lighting up her face. Relief washed over us as we realized that everything was alright; but we couldn't fully comprehend the magnitude of the news she was about to share.

In a moment that felt like an eternity, our doctor revealed that we were expecting not just one baby, but two babies—identical twins. Shock and overwhelming joy engulfed us, leaving us momentarily speechless. The doctor provided us with detailed instructions and guidance for a twin pregnancy, emphasizing the importance of extra care and vigilance.

It took us some time to truly grasp the reality of having two babies at once. The first part of our pregnancy was spent contemplating and wrapping our minds around the concept of becoming parents to twins. As the days passed, we shifted our focus to ensuring a healthy pregnancy, both physically and mentally. The second half of the pregnancy was dedicated to preparing my body and mind for a safe delivery and ensuring the well-being of our precious twins.

However, as I entered the third trimester, a new concern began to overshadow my thoughts. People around me, well-meaning friends and family, started expressing their opinions and suggesting a C-section for the delivery of the twins. Even our doctor seemed hesitant to provide a clear answer regarding the possibility of a vaginal delivery. This uncertainty left me feeling scared and stressed, groping for a definitive answer.

Approaching the 30-week mark of my pregnancy, the impending delivery weighed heavily on my mind. I longed for a sense of clarity, wanting to know if a twin pregnancy automatically meant a C-section. I yearned for a straightforward response that would allow me to prepare mentally and emotionally for the delivery. This constant uncertainty threatened to overshadow the joyous moments of my pregnancy journey.

Despite these concerns, I remind myself to embrace the beauty and blessings of carrying two precious lives within me. As I navigate the final weeks of my pregnancy, I strive to focus on staying healthy, nurturing my body, and trusting that the best course of action will become clearer as the delivery approaches. With the unwavering support of my husband and the guidance of medical professionals, I know that I can navigate the challenges and anxieties that come with a twin pregnancy.

HCG, or Human Chorionic Gonadotropin, is a hormone that is produced by the developing placenta after the fertilized egg attaches to the uterine lining. This typically occurs around 6 to 12 days after fertilization. The HCG hormone plays a vital role in supporting the production of progesterone and estrogen, which are necessary for thickening the uterine lining to support the growing embryo and maintain the pregnancy. Home pregnancy tests can detect the presence of HCG approximately two weeks after fertilization.

While every pregnancy and every woman is unique, HCG levels provide general statistics that help doctors assess the development of the pregnancy and the fetus. Typically, HCG hormone levels double every 72 hours after fertilization and reach their peak by the end of the first trimester. Afterward, they gradually decrease and stabilize for the remainder of the pregnancy. Monitoring the level of HCG in the blood can provide valuable information about the pregnancy and the health of the baby.

Higher levels of HCG can indicate a multiple pregnancy or abnormal growth in the uterus. Lower than expected levels may be indicative of a miscarriage or an increased risk of miscarriage. Slower than expected HCG level rise can suggest an ectopic pregnancy or other abnormalities, prompting the doctor to recommend an ultrasound to further investigate the situation.

A twin pregnancy, also known as a multiple pregnancy, can be influenced by both genetic and non-genetic factors. If twins run in your family, the likelihood of having twins increases. Additionally, the age of the woman plays a significant role, as older women are more likely to release more than one egg during ovulation. Fertility treatments such as in vitro fertilization (IVF) can also increase the chances of multiple pregnancies since multiple embryos may be transferred to the uterus to increase the chances of successful implantation.

Twins can be either monozygotic (identical twins) or dizygotic (fraternal twins). Monozygotic twins occur when a single fertilized egg splits into two embryos. These twins share identical DNA and are always of the same sex, exhibiting similar physical appearances and traits. The only distinguishing factor between identical twins is their fingerprints. While there may be similarities in the overall pattern, each individual has their own unique details and minutiae in their fingerprints. No two individuals have the exact same fingerprint in the world.

Dizygotic twins, on the other hand, are formed from two separate eggs that are fertilized by two different sperms. They do not share the same DNA and can be of the same sex or different sexes. These twins are siblings who shared the uterus simultaneously and are born at the same time.

Not all twin pregnancies are inherently complicated. It is possible to have a healthy twin pregnancy. However, having a twin pregnancy does increase the risk of certain complications and challenges, such as preterm birth, gestational diabetes, preeclampsia, twin-to-twin transfusion syndrome

(TTTS) in the case of identical twins, anemia, birth defects, miscarriage, postpartum hemorrhage, and the possibility of a C-section. Therefore, women with twin pregnancies require closer monitoring and more frequent prenatal visits to identify and address any potential complications.

However, it is important to note that not all twin pregnancies end in a C-section. The mode of delivery depends on various factors, including the position and size of the babies in the uterus, the progress of the pregnancy, and, most importantly, the health of the mother. The expertise and experience of the medical team also play a crucial role. Women with twin pregnancies should receive proper monitoring and regular consultations with their doctor to ensure appropriate care throughout their pregnancy journey.

Confronting the Fears of Maternity Leave: An Assurance to Working Mothers

At seven months pregnant, I found myself entangled in a web of emotions. A relentless workaholic, I had always been fiercely dedicated to my career, working tirelessly to reach the pinnacle of my profession. Although I was extremely excited about the impending arrival of my baby, I was also overcome with apprehension and uncertainty. The prospect of taking maternity leave was both thrilling and anxiety-inducing. My pregnancy had come as a surprise, adding yet another layer of complexity to the situation.

On one hand, I felt an intense longing to immerse myself in the journey of motherhood, to savor every moment of this miraculous new chapter in my life. I fantasized about cradling my baby, their delicate fingers clutching mine, their innocent gaze staring up at me. I yearned to cultivate a nurturing environment where love blossomed.

Yet, on the other hand, I was consumed by a gnawing anxiety about stepping away from my professional life. For years, my career had been a source of immense pride and satisfaction. It wasn't just a job to me—it was my purpose, my identity, an integral part of my existence. The thought of stepping back from it, even temporarily, felt akin to losing a part of myself. A chilling dread of becoming irrelevant in my professional realm haunted me relentlessly.

As I stood facing this transformative life event, I wrestled with unsettling questions. Would I lose my edge in the competitive corporate world? Would the ties I had painstakingly built with my peers and clients fray with my absence? The fear of falling behind, missing out on lucrative opportunities and key developments plagued me. But at the same time, the terror of missing out on my child's milestones, the small but monumental steps in their growth journey, weighed heavily on my heart.

Navigating this predicament felt like walking a tightrope with my heart pounding in my chest. Striking a balance between being a conscientious professional and a devoted mother seemed like an insurmountable task. I yearned to excel in my career while simultaneously witnessing every precious moment of my baby's development.

As my maternity leave approached, this internal struggle only intensified. The voice of reason reminded me to prioritize my health and my unborn child, but the siren call of my work and my ambition pulled me in the opposite direction. I felt as if I was standing at crossroads, with conflicting desires tugging me from either side.

Maternity leave is not an enjoyable or enviable period for many women. It has nothing to do with not wanting to be with your baby or not enjoying each and every second of the motherhood journey. Rather, it stems from the fear and uncertainty that arise when you step away from the career you have diligently built.

Questions and concerns flood your mind: What will happen during your absence? Will you be replaced? Will changes that occur while you're gone affect your position upon your return?

Let me assure you that your fears and doubts are completely valid and shared by countless women. Maternity changes numerous aspects of a woman's life, both physically and mentally, and has a profound impact on her professional and spiritual identity. It is natural to question your career path and contemplate the way you work. The uncertainty of how things may change can be overwhelming.

However, it is important to recognize that being on maternity leave does not diminish your skills or erase your past accomplishments. While you may miss out on certain opportunities or important events within your company, it is crucial to take it one step at a time. Embrace the fact that your working environment may need to be reorganized and that you may have to approach your career in a different way. This period can be viewed as a new chapter of your life—an opportunity to explore different avenues and discover new possibilities.

Remember, it's okay to go with the flow and allow yourself to be guided by the events of your life. Embrace the changes and challenges that come with motherhood, and trust in your ability to adapt and thrive. With time and patience, you will find your new rhythm and discover a balance that works for you and your growing family.

Overcoming Challenges: When Men Are Unwilling to Be Present at Childbirth

As my due date drew closer, the excitement became palpable in our cozy home in Mumbai. Our families—Rokith's and mine—eagerly awaited the arrival of our baby, who would be the first grandchild on both sides. The atmosphere was jubilant, and despite the occasional discomfort, my pregnancy had been a smooth sail.

One evening, with the aroma of home-cooked food filling the air, Rokith and I were immersed in an important discussion about the birth of our child. I had one earnest request: I wanted him to be there with me in the labor room during the birth.

Suddenly, as if a cloud had darkened his demeanor, Rokith's face contorted into a visage of sheer apprehension. It was as though an invisible barrier had risen between us. A tacit tradition within our family was that no man had ever stepped into the labor room. This was uncharted territory for him, and he seemed lost at sea with my request for his presence.

My heart swelled with an overwhelming deluge of emotions. This child was the living embodiment of our love, and I felt that Rokith's support in the labor room was an integral piece of the tapestry we were weaving together. I yearned for the steadiness of his hand and the solace of his whispers as I braced myself to bring our child into the world.

But as days slipped by, the house turned into a simmering cauldron of tension. Heated arguments ensued, and our voices reverberated through the halls like clashing waves. Each exchange was like a splinter in the fabric of our relationship. His reservations, in stark contrast to my longing, left me grappling to understand him; yet every night brought no solace, only a growing chasm.

My mother-in-law, ever the bedrock of the family, saw the turmoil raging within me. Although her words were soothing as a balm, they could not quell the storm that was brewing between Rokith and me.

Night after night, as I lay awake, I wrestled with his perspective, attempting to penetrate the fog of his apprehensions. However, an undercurrent of frustration and disenchantment continued to shroud my soul. The very thought of him not wanting to be there at the pinnacle of our shared journey felt like a betrayal.

The echoes of our arguments and the cold silences that followed, continued to strain the bond that had once seemed unbreakable. It was as if an invisible wedge had been driven between us, and I feared the rift would only widen as the delivery day drew closer.

After wrestling with my feelings for a while, I decided that it was time to have an open, candid conversation with my partner. It was not just about my needs, but about our journey as a couple, as parents-to-be. Under the starlit night, I poured my heart out to Rokith. My voice quivered as I explained how his support meant the world to me and how sharing this transformative experience could strengthen the bond we cherished. "We're in this together," I whispered.

Eventually, we had an open discussion about our feelings and concerns, unraveling the layers of our hearts and connecting on a deeper level. In that space of honesty and vulnerability, we discovered a newfound strength, a unity that would carry us through the highs and lows of parenthood.

Contrary to how it may seem, this is a rather common predicament. For women, it's an unavoidable sense of injustice. Women shoulder the bulk of the physical burden, when it comes to birthing a baby. The discomfort, the pain, and the act of birthing itself, are endured by the woman alone. From the man's perspective, however, the situation may seem dauntingly unbalanced.

The labor room is far from a serene haven. There will be blood, bodily fluids, noise, screaming, and a flurry of medical professionals. The sight of their partner in pain can be unbearable for some men. Many men experience a feeling of helplessness as they stand by, unable to alleviate their partner's suffering. Others may have an aversion to the sight of blood or medical procedures, which can trigger feelings of nausea or unease.

As much as these reasons might seem valid, they can cause feelings of abandonment and lack of support in the woman. She may carry these feelings long after the birth, which could potentially strain the relationship. Therefore, it is crucial to discuss this issue early on, aiming for a mutual understanding.

Even after several discussions, if the man is unwilling to change his stance, his feelings must be respected. However, no woman should endure labor and its associated pain alone. It is essential to have someone who can offer emotional support, other than a medical professional. This support person, be it a relative or a friend or a doula, can assist with pain management techniques and provide comfort during labor.

Labor preparation classes can be extremely beneficial in preparing the support person for their role. Their contribution is critical for the progress and duration of labor. While the situation might seem challenging, it is just one of the many hurdles that you will cross in this beautiful journey toward parenthood. As you grapple with the complexities of this issue, always remember to trust your instincts, communicate openly, and ensure your comfort and well-being during this transformative phase.

Your Body, Your Choice: Asserting Autonomy in Childbirth

As I reached the ninth month of my unexpected but cherished pregnancy, a mix of joy and anticipation filled my heart. I, Rahini, a woman who had always been independent and determined, was about to embark on an incredible journey—motherhood. The thought of my body preparing to bring a new life into the world was both awe-inspiring and humbling.

Driven by my natural inclination to be informed and proactive, I absorbed as much knowledge as I could about my pregnancy. Prenatal yoga, nourishing meals, and hours of research on childbirth became a part of my routine. I felt a deep sense of purpose, a strong desire to approach this chapter of my life with awareness and confidence. I had made a decision—I wanted to experience labor without medical interventions, trusting in the strength of my body.

This desire was not a passing fancy; it was rooted in my deep understanding of myself and my capabilities. I wanted to be fully present for every moment of this incredible journey.

However, when I shared my wish with my doctor, her response was far from supportive. She dismissed my desire for an unmedicated delivery, reasoning that many women ultimately requested pain relief. Her lack of faith in my choice sent shockwaves through me. Even my partner, Vivek, expressed doubts. It seemed that my family, whom I had hoped would be my biggest support, also questioned my decision.

But their skepticism only fueled my determination. I knew that choosing an unmedicated birth was not a whim; it was a well-considered choice, grounded in my own knowledge and beliefs.

To find solace and guidance, I reached out to other women who had experienced unmedicated births. Their stories became my refuge; their experiences became a guiding light in the darkness of doubt. They showed me that it was possible to navigate labor without medical interventions and emerge stronger from it.

With their support, I delved deeper into preparing myself mentally and physically for the journey ahead. I practiced relaxation techniques and focused on my well-being, knowing that a calm mind and body would be paramount for a smooth labor.

I refused to let the doubts and criticisms discourage me. I stood my ground and defended my choice to my family. It wasn't just about having an unmedicated birth; it was about asserting my autonomy as a woman and embracing the right to make decisions about my own body and birthing experience.

The journey of pregnancy and childbirth is monumental for a couple, but more so for a woman. It is a transformative phase that changes her life and her body in ways unimaginable. It is only fair that a woman's desires and concerns take center stage when it comes to childbirth. Therefore, the decision of how she brings a new life into the world should be hers to make.

Unfortunately, in many cultures, doctors often hold an unquestionable authority. They are seen as infallible, their words treated as gospel truth.

This perception needs to evolve with time. Doctors are human, prone to the same biases and conditioned thinking as the rest of us. It's time we stopped placing them on a pedestal, especially when it comes to childbirth.

The medical landscape has been changing significantly, with several options available for pain management during labor, including water births, and the support of a doula during delivery. The choice of the doctor and hospital plays a critical role in how a woman experiences her pregnancy and delivery. It's important that these choices align with her desires, supporting her as she navigates this life-changing journey.

Educating oneself about these options and asserting one's choice is paramount. But equally important is having the support of one's partner and family during this time. If faced with resistance, it is essential to articulate your needs and decisions assertively, as I did. Pregnancy and childbirth are as much about mental strength as physical, and having your loved ones understand and support your choices is invaluable.

Navigating Sleep Disruptions During Pregnancy

My name is Kavitha, and I am currently 34 weeks pregnant. This pregnancy was unexpected; but although we didn't plan to have a baby, we are overjoyed and excited for our little one's arrival. However, as the weeks progress, I find myself growing tired and longing for the pregnancy to come to an end soon.

From the very beginning, my pregnancy has been challenging. As a freelancer, I have the flexibility to manage my work and personal time. Usually, I enjoy indulging in my hobbies and, most of all, sleeping, because I love it so much. But since the start of my pregnancy, getting a proper night's sleep has been elusive. The constant fatigue has taken a toll on me, leaving me tired all the time, even after what should have been a good night's rest.

During the first trimester, I experienced nausea, vomiting, and extreme tiredness. I constantly felt drained and lacked the refreshing feeling that sleep should provide. Being caught off guard by this pregnancy has also made me anxious. Questions flood my mind all the time: What will life be like after the baby is born? Will I be a good mother? Will I understand and meet my baby's needs? What if something goes wrong during labor? These uncertainties keep me restless, making it even more difficult to sleep.

As I entered the second trimester, heartburn and frequent trips to the bathroom added to my sleep woes. And now, leg cramps have joined the list of discomforts. Despite all these challenges, when I do manage to fall asleep, vivid dreams plague my nights. It feels like my fears and worries manifest in my dreams, further hindering the quality of my rest.

For someone who cherishes sleep, not getting enough of it has been incredibly frustrating and irritating. It's disheartening to feel tired all the time, and this exhaustion often transforms into irritability, leading to arguments with my husband or family members. Knowing that in a few weeks, I will have a baby to care for only adds to my apprehension, as I anticipate more sleepless nights due to feeding and tending to my little one's needs. I feel exhausted and helpless.

However, amid the fatigue and challenges, I try to remind myself that this is just a temporary phase. As I navigate these final weeks of pregnancy, I hold on to the hope that once my baby arrives, the exhaustion will be worth it, and a new chapter of joy and fulfillment will begin.

We all know that pregnancy comes with its benefits and discomforts. While many people talk about the common symptoms like nausea, vomiting, and back pain, not enough attention is given to sleep problems during pregnancy. Yet, changes in sleep patterns are quite common throughout the journey of pregnancy. During the first trimester, you may notice a shift in your sleeping patterns—feeling slightly drowsier than usual or experiencing increased fatigue. Other discomforts such as heartburn, leg pain, frequent trips to the bathroom, and back pain can also influence the quality of your sleep. Additionally, the combination of hormonal changes, physical discomfort, extreme tiredness, fear of labor and childbirth, and the anticipation of becoming a mother can cause vivid and sometimes strange dreams.

Tiredness and sleep problems, including insomnia, can have a significant impact on both your health and your pregnancy. Quality sleep is essential for allowing your body to rest, recharge, stabilize blood sugar levels, and support a strong immune system. Sleep also plays a crucial role in memory, learning, appetite, mood, and decision-making. Sleep deprivation can affect both maternal and fetal health.

Fortunately, you can improve the quality of your sleep by making slight adjustments to your lifestyle:

Address other discomforts: *Take steps to alleviate discomforts that may be affecting your sleep. For example, if frequent trips to the bathroom disrupt your sleep, try drinking plenty of fluids throughout the day but reducing fluid intake closer to bedtime. Use dim lighting in your bedroom and bathroom during nighttime visits to make it easier to return to sleep.*

Manage heartburn: *Pregnancy hormones can cause muscles to relax, including those that normally keep the stomach acid in the stomach. This relaxation, combined with the growing uterus pressing on the abdomen, can worsen heartburn. To manage heartburn, avoid spicy foods, eat smaller meals, have dinner at least two hours before bed, elevate your head with a few pillows, and sleep on your left side. If heartburn becomes intolerable, consult your doctor for further guidance.*

Deal with nasal congestion: *Hormonal changes during pregnancy increase blood volume throughout the body, leading to swollen nasal membranes and increased mucus production, resulting in nasal congestion. Elevating your head with a few pillows can help alleviate the congestion. Consult your doctor for appropriate treatment options.*

Adjust your lifestyle: *Make some lifestyle changes to promote better sleep. Avoid screen time before bed, limit caffeine intake in the* *evening, engage in daily physical activity, have an early dinner, establish a bedtime routine, practice breathing exercises or meditation, and consider maintaining a journal to write down your thoughts, fears, and doubts. Journaling can help manage anxiety and promote a sense of calm before sleep. If sleep deprivation continues to be a problem in your daily life, don't hesitate to discuss it with your doctor.*

By addressing discomforts, making lifestyle adjustments, and seeking appropriate guidance, you can improve your sleep quality during pregnancy. Remember that taking care of your sleep is essential for your well-being and the health of both you and your baby.

Breech Presentation: Navigating Your Options

My name is Maya, and I'm a professor. I'm an organized and anticipated person, someone who appreciates when things go according to plan. When I found out I was pregnant, it was unexpected but nonetheless exciting. Throughout my pregnancy, I experienced minimal discomfort—just some fatigue and occasional back pain. Overall, it was an uncomplicated, happy, and relatively easy pregnancy.

My husband and I were fully invested in this journey together. We attended prenatal classes and diligently prepared ourselves mentally and physically for the upcoming birth. It was a beautiful time for us, filled with anticipation and joy. However, during a routine check-up scan around 32 weeks, the doctor mentioned that our baby had not turned head down yet. At the time, the doctor assured us that there was still time and that some babies turn head down a bit later. So, we didn't think much of it and continued with our preparations.

Fast forward to the 34-week scan, and the baby was still not in the head down position. This time, the doctor discussed the possibility of an eventual C-section if the baby didn't turn on their own before the due date. The news caught us off guard, as I wasn't mentally prepared for the possibility of a C-section. I had been so focused on preparing for a vaginal delivery that this sudden change of plans was a jolt to my expectations.

During our prenatal classes, we had learned about the importance of the optimal position for a vaginal birth, and I remembered a few exercises and techniques that could potentially help the baby turn head down. I tried everything—yoga, breathing exercises, specific positions, and movements—but nothing seemed to work. As my due date approached, the baby remained in a breech position, and the doctor informed me that a C-section would be necessary if the baby didn't turn by 40 weeks.

I felt a mix of disappointment and acceptance. Despite all my efforts, if the baby didn't turn, then it was meant to be this way. I shifted my mindset to focus on having a positive birthing experience, regardless of the mode of delivery. With that in mind, I decided to attend a preparation class specifically for C-section. This class provided valuable insights into the procedure and helped me prepare mentally for what was to come.

Two days after my due date, my beautiful baby girl was born via C-section. Despite initially feeling disappointed about not having a vaginal birth, I can genuinely say that I had a positive birthing experience. My doctor was incredibly compassionate and understanding throughout the process. She gave me the time and space to adapt to this new plan, explaining everything thoroughly and simply being there for me. In her care, I felt understood and empowered.

This experience taught me that a C-section birth can also be positive. What truly matters is how you feel during the birth—whether you feel supported, understood, and empowered.

A breech presentation occurs when the baby's feet or buttocks are positioned on the cervix, ready to come out first instead of the head. Most babies naturally turn head down around 36 weeks, assuming a vertex presentation, which is the optimal position for birth. However, around 3 to 4 percent of babies remain in a breech position by the end of pregnancy.

There are different types of breech positions. The first is the Frank breech, where the baby's buttocks are on the cervix, and the feet are near the head, somewhat resembling the "happy baby" yoga position. The second is the complete breech, where the baby's buttocks are still on the cervix, with the legs folded at the knees and the feet near the buttocks, akin to sitting cross-legged on the floor. The third type is the footling breech, where one or both of the baby's feet point toward the birth canal to come out first.

The exact cause of breech presentation is not fully understood; but certain factors can influence this positioning. These factors include the level of amniotic fluid, abnormalities in the shape of the uterus or abnormal growths such as fibroids, placenta previa (where the placenta completely covers the opening of the uterus), multiple pregnancies, and a history of premature delivery.

It is important to note that breech presentation does not always indicate complications or an unhealthy baby. Various techniques can be attempted to turn a breech baby; but it's crucial to discuss the options with your doctor to determine which method may be suitable for you.

One non-surgical method is External Cephalic Version (ECV), where the baby is manually turned from the outside. This procedure is performed by experienced professionals while closely monitoring the mother. Like any medical procedure, ECV carries its own risks, such as placental abruption, preterm delivery, rupture of membranes, or changes in fetal heart rate. The process can be uncomfortable or even painful for some women. However, ECV is not appropriate for everyone, particularly those with multiple pregnancies or low amniotic fluid levels.

Other methods to encourage the baby to turn include specific exercises, hot and cold packs, sound therapy, meditation, and breathing techniques. While the efficacy of these methods requires further research, they are generally safe for you and your baby. However, it is crucial to consult your doctor for guidance and determine the best course of action.

It's important to note that a breech presentation does not always necessitate a C-section. The choice of a vaginal delivery depends on several factors, including the baby's position (which specific breech position the baby is in), the baby's health, the baby's weight to ensure safe passage through the birth canal, and the experience and comfort level of the medical team in performing a breech vaginal delivery.

The main risk associated with a breech vaginal delivery is the potential for the body to deliver while the head remains stuck within the cervix, as the baby's head is the last part to come out. Another complication is cord prolapse, where the umbilical cord gets compressed as the baby moves toward the birth canal, potentially reducing oxygen and blood flow.

Due to these risks, most doctors recommend a C-section for breech presentation babies. However, discussing your specific circumstances with your doctor is essential to determine the safest and most appropriate delivery option for you and your baby.

Understanding and Embracing Authority in your Birthing Journey

For an entrepreneur like me, life is like a whirlwind, and I, Pragathi, have always been at the center, following the tunes of innovation and ambition. So, when I discovered that a little one was growing within me, it felt like nature had gracefully woven itself into the fabric of my fast-paced life. My partner, Sathish, and I embraced this journey with all the wisdom we could muster.

As I walked into the doctor's office, each step felt heavy with the culmination of a thorough search for the perfect healthcare provider. Sathish and I had painstakingly sought opinions and recommendations before zeroing in on a reputable doctor and hospital that we believed would make our journey as prospective parents smooth. The anticipation of meeting our little one made the series of brief, 5–10 minute appointments seem worthwhile, as we felt secure about our choice.

However, life, with its propensity for unpredictability, had other plans. In the final leg of my pregnancy, the doctor informed me that my amniotic fluid was low, and prescribed a supplement. I took it religiously for weeks, eager to do anything necessary for the well-being of our baby. On what was supposed to be a routine visit following a busy day at work, I settled in for my prenatal appointment.

As I composed myself, my doctor casually mentioned that she had performed a membrane sweep due to low amniotic fluid levels. She reassured me that a vaginal delivery was still possible and then asked me to take an ultrasound at an external scan center to confirm the amniotic fluid levels. I was blindsided and shell-shocked; I couldn't muster the words to ask her why she had taken this step without informing me.

Emotions cascaded through me like a torrential downpour—anger, betrayal, fear, and anxiety engulfed me as I rushed to an external scan center. However, the scan results baffled me—it revealed that my amniotic fluid levels were perfectly normal. The dam of emotions broke. I felt deceived. Trust was shattered, and the plans we had laid out with so much hope seemed to crumble before our eyes.

Sathish and I, still reeling, realized how profoundly a doctor's actions can impact an expectant mother's pregnancy journey. We made the difficult decision to change both the hospital and the doctor. My faith was shaken, but with the unyielding support of my husband, I garnered the strength to move forward.

I had envisioned the third trimester to be a nurturing phase, a time to create a cozy home for our baby and indulge in baby shopping. It was meant to be a period of daydreaming about how our lives would transform. However, we ended up going through the turmoil of finding a new doctor at this crucial juncture of my pregnancy.

Ultimately, we found a good doctor and I had a vaginal delivery; but the harrowing experience with the first doctor left an indelible mark on me. It served as a reminder of the importance of compassion, transparency, and trust in the delicate tapestry of bringing a new life into the world.

Imagine this scenario: You are nearing the final stages of your pregnancy, eagerly anticipating the moment when you will cradle your precious newborn in your arms. However, amid your excitement, your healthcare provider mentions a procedure called "membrane sweep." Your brows furrow in confusion. What precisely does this entail?

Allow me to shed some light on the matter, articulating the details. Consider the membrane sweep as a gentle nudge on your baby, urging them to embrace the world beyond the womb. In this procedure, the skilled hands of your healthcare provider would use a gloved finger to separate the amniotic sac from the walls of the uterus. While this may not be the most glamorous experience, rest assured, it is a common procedure that is done on many expectant mothers.

Now, you may wonder, what purpose does this serve? Think of it as an ignition spark to revitalize a dormant engine. When the membrane sweep is done, your body receives a signal to produce labor hormones, ushering the onset of childbirth. It is a natural approach, devoid of medicinal intervention. One minor downside of this procedure is that it may elicit certain unfamiliar sensations, such as some light bleeding, contractions, cramping, or mild discomfort. But there will be no risk for the baby.

However, here's the clincher—there are instances when your body may not respond to the initial sweep. In such cases, your healthcare provider may need to repeat the procedure. If your body still remains unresponsive, they may resort to more assertive measures, such as breaking the water bag or administering medications to induce labor. While the sweep serves as an opening act, the main event may require a more forceful push.

Now, take a moment to catch your breath. I understand that this information may be overwhelming. However, remember that you hold the reins of your pregnancy journey. You possess the authority to seek clarification, pose inquiries, and ensure that your needs are met. You are the protagonist in this narrative, an empowered individual, entrusted with safeguarding the well-being of both yourself and your precious child.

It is imperative to recognize that as a patient, especially an expectant mother, you should be informed and asked for consent before any medical procedure is conducted—be it a membrane sweep, ultrasound, vaccination, or even something as mundane as a urine sample test. This holds true regardless of the stage of your pregnancy. Patient consent is a fundamental cornerstone of medical ethics and practice.

Should any concerns arise or should you find that your rapport with your healthcare provider or chosen medical facility is not aligned, remember that you possess the agency to seek alternative options. This decision carries great weight, transcending mere choices of convenience or preference.

And let us not forget the fundamental principle that knowledge is empowering. The more you acquaint yourself with the subject at hand, the more informed decisions you can make for the benefit of yourself and your unborn child.

Prepare yourself, for you are a formidable force, a warrior in this extraordinary journey. Equip yourself with knowledge, pose those pertinent questions, and brace yourself to welcome your little one with wisdom and confidence.

Preparation and Pain Management During Labor: A Balanced Perspective

My name is Leela, and I live in Bangalore with my husband, Maran. Our pregnancy journey was a mix of excitement and conscious preparation. Although it wasn't a planned pregnancy, we were overjoyed when we found out that we were expecting. From the very beginning, we made it a priority to educate ourselves about pregnancy and childbirth. Attending prenatal classes and engaging in discussions with healthcare professionals became a regular part of our routine.

As the months went by, I developed a strong desire for an unmedicated delivery. I wanted to experience the rawness and empowerment of bringing my baby into the world naturally. I diligently practiced various exercises and breathing techniques that would help me cope with the intensity of labor. With each passing day, I gained not only physical endurance but also mental strength in preparation for the big day.

However, when labor finally began, I quickly realized that the pain was far beyond what I had imagined. The intensity was unbearable, even with the comfort measures and coping techniques that I had learned. After hours of enduring the excruciating pain, I made the difficult decision to request an epidural. The medical team promptly responded and the relief it provided allowed me to take a breather.

But amid the relief, I couldn't shake off the feeling of disappointment and failure. The longing for an unmedicated birth still lingered within me. Even three months postpartum, the guilt of not having followed through with my original plan weighs heavily on my heart. I often question myself if I should have persevered and pushed through the pain to achieve the unmedicated birth that I had envisioned.

It's a complex mix of emotions. On one hand, I am immensely grateful for the safe arrival of my precious baby. On the other hand, I can't help but feel a sense of personal failure for not having achieved what I had set out to do. The journey of motherhood has taught me that birth plans don't always unfold as expected, and it's important to be gentle with ourselves and embrace the choices we make during such a vulnerable time.

Sharing my story is my way of processing these emotions and hopefully connecting with others who have experienced similar feelings.

Labor is a natural process, and our bodies are designed to give birth in a natural way. However, in today's modern world, we have options for pain management during labor. These options include epidurals, nitrous oxide/Entonox, and painkiller injections, among others. Apart from these medical interventions, there are also natural pain management techniques such as breathing exercises, certain positions, movements, and massages that can be beneficial. It is important to start preparing for labor early in pregnancy and continue the preparation until delivery in order to reap the benefits of your preparation.

Even if you are planning to have an epidural or other medication to manage pain during labor, it is crucial to also prepare yourself for an unmedicated delivery. This is because labor can be quite unpredictable. You may face a situation in which pain medication is not an option. Your doctor might advise against it, the epidural might not work effectively, or you may not have sufficient time to receive the medication. Therefore, being mentally and physically prepared to manage pain without medication is essential. Additionally, recovery from an unmedicated delivery tends to be faster.

It is important to remember that every woman is different, and pain tolerance varies from person to person. Until you are in labor, you cannot truly know how painful it will be or whether you will be able to handle it without medication. It is not a reflection of failure if you choose or need to have a medicated delivery. There are no rules stating that you must endure the pain until the end or prove anything to anyone.

Each individual has their own limit of pain tolerance, and respecting your own boundaries is key. The most important thing is to have a safe and healthy birthing experience, regardless of the pain management approach chosen. The emphasis is to ensure that the experience is empowering and positive, irrespective of the path taken. By focusing on the health and well-being of both the mother and the child, and by making choices that respect one's own limits and needs, the birthing experience can be made into a cherished memory that is enveloped in love and strength.

Inside the Womb: Dealing with Low Amniotic Fluid During Pregnancy

I am Gayathri, a mother of a 4-month-old baby boy. When I learned that I was expecting, my heart overflowed with joy. This child was dearly awaited by my husband and me. Our dreams were taking shape and the future seemed full of promise.

My pregnancy progressed smoothly and I savored each moment of it. However, the 20-week scan did not go quite as expected. My husband couldn't accompany me on that day as he had an important commitment. So I went alone, expecting it to be another routine appointment. However, what happened at the hospital was quite out of routine. The lab doctors seemed more attentive than usual, scanning and re-scanning. I was asked to wait for the consulting gynecologist. As the minutes ticked by, my heart raced; something felt amiss.

Finally, the gynecologist arrived and called me in. The grave look on her face worried me. She gently explained that my amniotic fluid levels were lower than normal, which could have adverse consequences on my baby's growth and well-being. My mind fixated on the words "lower than normal," and the room began to spin. My husband arrived just in time to catch the doctor's detailed instructions. All I could process was a mixture of worry and disbelief.

Days turned into weeks, and my routine was tightly scheduled around monitoring and tests. My doctor urged me to drink water relentlessly and cut back on physical activity. I had to rest, be calm, and stay hydrated. Moreover, my sugar levels were elevated. My emotions were on a roller coaster, and all I wanted was to ensure the safety of my unborn child.

The 30th week scan indicated that my amniotic fluid levels still remained low. My doctor, being my guardian angel, guided me through these tough times to the maximum extent possible. I spent my days on pins and needles, feeling helpless yet willing to do anything within my means to protect my baby.

When I reached 34 weeks, my doctor decided that it was time for me to get admitted to the hospital. My amniotic fluid was decreasing, and she did not want to take any chances. I was put on bed rest, and the ensuing days felt like an eternity.

As the delivery date drew near, my doctor advised that it was best for the baby to be born sooner rather than later. A discussion ensued about inducing labor to allow for a vaginal birth. My heart yearned for a natural delivery, but I was well aware that we might have to go in for a C-section if my body didn't respond to the medications as expected. The doctor left no stone unturned, explaining all the risks involved and giving us ample time to decide. Finally, we decided to go in for induced labor.

Medications for inducing labor were administered and then, like a miracle, my body responded. My precious baby boy was born through a vaginal delivery. However, he was slightly underweight and had to spend three to four weeks in the NICU to get strong enough for life outside my womb.

Now, as I hold my healthy and happy baby in my arms, gratitude fills my soul. I am immensely indebted to the medical team and my doctor, who helped us navigate through the storm with grace and commitment. The journey was far from easy, but every second was worth it for the gift that is my son.

The amniotic fluid, which cradles your baby in the womb, is a vital component in your pregnancy journey. Ensconced within the amniotic sac, this fluid cushions your baby, facilitating movements and fostering the development of vital organs, such as the lungs and kidneys. Furthermore, it safeguards the umbilical cord from getting compressed by the uterus.

However, sometimes there may be a dip in the amniotic fluid level, resulting in a condition known as "oligohydramnios." This may happen due to a variety of reasons, including premature rupture of membranes, placental abruption, anomalies in the baby's kidney or urinary tract, pre-existing maternal health conditions, dehydration, or overdue pregnancies.

Here is an interesting fact: The amniotic fluid, which is mainly sourced from your body, starts forming about 12 days after conception. Post 20 weeks of pregnancy, the baby's urine replenishes the fluid. Rich in nutrients, hormones, and antibodies, the fluid peaks around the 36th week, then gradually decreases until delivery.

Oligohydramnios can lead to potential complications for the baby, such as preterm birth, growth retardation, and in rare instances, stillbirth. It may also cause the baby to inhale their first stool, known as meconium, into their lungs.

Oligohydramnios is usually detected through ultrasound measurements or by identifying premature rupture of membranes. The method of treating this condition will vary based on the stage of pregnancy and associated complications. If the pregnancy is near-term, inducing labor might be the chosen path to avoid complications. Otherwise, you can expect actions such as close monitoring, frequent check-ups, and tests.

While it is critical for your baby to grow and develop fully before birth, treatments for oligohydramnios will be tailored based on individual symptoms and health conditions of the mother and the baby, among other factors. Doctors may advise drinking ample water, resting, reducing physical activities, and constant monitoring.

This condition can be prevented by having regular prenatal check-ups, remaining hydrated, and following a healthy diet. Although oligohydramnios is a significant health concern, it is important to remember that many babies diagnosed with low amniotic fluid go on to be born healthy. So, while vigilance is necessary, undue stress should be avoided.

Postpartum Period

Beyond Childbirth: The Overlooked Reality of Postpartum

The news of our much-anticipated pregnancy filled our hearts with an indescribable joy. We had been longing for this moment, and when we discovered that I was expecting, it felt like a dream come true. Throughout my pregnancy, we took every step necessary to ensure a smooth journey. Attending prenatal classes and educating ourselves about postpartum care, breastfeeding, and newborn care made us feel prepared for what lay ahead. With the unwavering support of both our families, I felt confident that the postpartum phase would be manageable.

Little did I know that I was about to embark on one of the most challenging periods of my life. The moment my baby entered the world, an incredible surge of hormones took hold, and my body underwent a profound transformation. It was as if a switch had been flipped, and suddenly, I found myself facing a daunting combination of sleepless nights, overwhelming anxiety, and heightened vigilance. The weight of baby blues and the dark cloud of postpartum depression descended upon me, casting a shadow on what should have been a blissful time.

I found myself grappling with emotions I had never experienced before. The constant hormonal fluctuations and the exhaustion took a toll on my mental and emotional well-being. There were moments when the overwhelming intensity of it all made me yearn for a break, for a reprieve from the relentless demands of motherhood. I loved my baby with all my heart, but there were times when I questioned my ability to navigate this new chapter of my life.

In the depths of postpartum depression, it felt like I was trapped between two conflicting worlds. On one hand, I longed to be fully present for my precious bundle of joy, cherishing every moment of her growth. On the other hand, I couldn't shake off the persistent feeling of wanting to escape, to find solace in a space where the weight of my emotions didn't consume me. It was a complex and overwhelming mix of emotions, one that left me feeling raw and vulnerable.

Yet, amid the darkness, a glimmer of hope emerged. With the support of my loved ones, I found the courage to reach out for help. Through therapy, self-care practices, and the unwavering love and understanding of my partner and family, I started to find my way back to a place of balance and healing. Each step forward was celebrated with small victories, and I began to see glimpses of light breaking through the clouds.

This journey through postpartum depression has taught me the importance of self-compassion, seeking support, and embracing the imperfections of motherhood. I am learning to be gentle with myself, acknowledging that it's okay to not have all the answers and to ask for help when needed. My love for my baby remains unwavering, and I am determined to provide her with the best version of myself.

Postpartum is a phase that is often overlooked and underestimated in discussions surrounding pregnancy and childbirth. In our culture, the postpartum period focuses primarily on the physical aspects, with an emphasis on providing good food and rest for the mother. Unfortunately, mental well-being is often neglected or dismissed. It is commonly believed that having a baby and a supportive family, along with good food, should be enough to make a woman happy. Any mention of anxiety, tears, or a lack of enthusiasm for baby care may be met with disbelief or even judgment.

However, postpartum is a real and significant period. In medical terms, it encompasses the first six months after delivery, which is the approximate time the body takes to recover from childbirth. It is important to note that every woman and each delivery is unique, so this is only an average timeframe. During this phase, it is normal to experience feelings of loneliness, fatigue, irritability, and even mild mood swings. Your body has undergone significant hormonal changes throughout pregnancy, and after delivery, these hormone levels rapidly decrease. This sudden hormonal shift can make women more susceptible to mood swings and heightened sensitivity. This is commonly known as "baby blues," and affects approximately 80% of new mothers.

Postpartum depression occurs when feelings of depression, persistent mood swings, sadness, or even thoughts of harming oneself or the baby persist for an extended period. If you experience these symptoms, it is crucial to consult your doctor for appropriate support and guidance. It is important to understand that feelings of depression, loneliness, irritability, or being easily overwhelmed are quite common during the postpartum period.

Motherhood can often feel lonely and challenging, but it is undoubtedly a worthwhile journey. For me, the postpartum period extended beyond the standard six months or one year; it encompassed three years. Many countries recognize this extended timeframe, as it takes a significant amount of time for a mother to navigate through baby care, breastfeeding, diaper changes, and gradually find her sense of self again. It can be difficult to leave the baby without worrying, and it often takes three years for a mother to regain a sense of balance and autonomy in her life.

It is crucial to seek help and support to navigate this postpartum period. Don't hesitate to reach out to your partner, family, and friends for assistance. Take small breaks throughout the day to catch your breath, indulge in activities you enjoy, or simply rest. Opening up about your feelings and concerns with someone you trust can be incredibly therapeutic. Consider writing a journal to express your thoughts and emotions. Remember, this phase is temporary; it's a time of learning, challenges, doubts, and tears; but it's also a time for unconditional love, hugs, kisses, and magical moments. It's a journey that is undeniably worth it.

Reclaiming Motherhood: Negotiating Space in a Traditional Landscape

As Laxmy, I held my precious Nakshathra in my arms, stepping into a world of dreams. Her soft cheeks and tiny fingers filled my heart with love. I was excited to be a mother and cherished every moment of motherhood. But amid all the joy, challenges started emerging.

Living with my family, I expected support and comfort. However, well-meaning relatives often took Nakshathra away, leaving me longing to hold her, to be her safe place. Their comments and judgment made me feel inadequate, like I did not know how to be a mother.

Nadesh, my husband, could only be with us on weekends, and I sometimes felt lost without him. I wanted to tell everyone, "Let me learn what makes my baby happy. Let me be the one she turns to."

Instead of finding the support I hoped for, I felt isolated. It was as if I was watching Nakshathra from a distance, unable to fully guide and nurture her. I wished for the strength to embrace motherhood on my own terms, to trust my instincts.

The constant scrutiny was frustrating and overwhelming, to say the least. I was reduced from the primary caregiver to a subject of critique. My confidence was eroding, my role as a mother seemingly diminishing under the weight of everyone else's opinion.

What worsened the situation was the unintentional intrusion into my bonding time with my baby. Well-intentioned family members would often swoop in after her feeding times, and whisk her away for playtime. I felt sidelined, like a spectator of my own child's growing days. I yearned for those intimate moments of connection with my newborn, the quiet lullabies, and gentle cuddles—the simple pleasures of motherhood that I was being deprived of.

I was the one who had carried her for nine months and endured the trials of labor but yet, it felt like I was being reduced to a mere feeder. I craved the liberty to care for my child, to experience the highs and lows of her growth journey without constant interference.

Laxmy's sentiment resonates with that of many first-time mothers, especially when their baby is the first in the family. It is common to feel like a "feeding station," a role that barely scratches the surface of what motherhood entails. Tradition often dictates that the elders in the family take over the responsibilities of newborn care. They do this out of love, and perhaps habit, for it was their mothers or mothers-in-law who did the same for them.

These generational differences often create misunderstandings. Modern mothers crave to spend time with their babies, savoring every moment and making every decision that affects the baby. Meanwhile, elders in the family, acting out of concern, often believe that by taking over some responsibilities, they are allowing the new mother to rest and recover.

There is a unique bond between a mother and her baby, a primal instinct that is deeply ingrained in us. The desire to protect our young, to be close, to smell and touch them, is intrinsic to our nature. This innate connection often manifests in seemingly unusual ways. For instance, a baby may appear calm and playful with everyone else, but the moment they are back in their mother's arms, they might start crying. This is because a mother is a child's sanctuary—the one place where they can freely express their emotions without fear or inhibition.

These initial phases of motherhood can feel isolating. It's a struggle to balance the joy of nurturing your child with the challenges of living up to the expectations of others. However, it is crucial to remember that you, as a mother, have an intimate bond with your baby. You should feel empowered to shape this relationship in a manner that respects your instincts and caters to your baby's needs. Conversations can go a long way in bridging this gap—express your feelings, assert your role as a mother, and negotiate the space you need with your baby. Motherhood is a unique journey, one that should be cherished, not overshadowed by unwarranted pressures.

Matrescence: Understanding the Transformation into Motherhood

I am Tara, a new mother. Four months ago, when I held my little bundle of joy, my son Rishi, in my arms for the first time, emotions surged through me like a tidal wave. The hospital room was imbued with the intoxicating essence of new beginnings. The world seemed to have dawned anew, painted in hues I had never seen before. But within this cascade of joy, a soft tune of worries began to hum in my mind.

As I gingerly crossed the threshold into our home, holding Rishi close to my heart, the walls seemed to whisper stories of generations of mothers who had walked this path before me. Their silent tales enveloped me, and I was swept into a tempest of thoughts.

The echoing whispers grew louder, but they were my own. "Is Rishi okay?", "Am I doing this right?", "What if I'm not enough?" The litany of questions roared like an incessant storm. Rishi's gentle breaths were a soft lullaby that struggled against the crescendo of self-doubt that threatened to overpower me.

Did everyone have the answers but me? Was there a secret script to motherhood that I had not been given? The weight of every tear that slipped from Rishi's eyes seemed like an indication of my poor mothering abilities. Every cry felt like an accusation, a stern finger pointing at my inexperience and questioning my competence.

As days turned into weeks, I found myself struggling to navigate the rocky terrain of motherhood. I was wracked with physical exhaustion from sleepless nights and the persistent needs of my tiny human. However, it was the emotional toll that took me by surprise. The endless sea of questions, the self-imposed scrutiny, and the incessant dissection of my every move formed a vortex that threatened to engulf me. The nagging voice inside me that whispered, "Are you sure?" never seemed to fade.

I desperately wanted to be a good mother. The kind that could weather any storm with grace. But the specter of my own expectations haunted me. Each day was a gauntlet, testing the mettle of my resolve.

I knew I needed to find a balance, to calm the storm within. This journey, I realized, was not just about protecting and nurturing Rishi; it was also about protecting and nurturing myself.

As the months rolled on, my confidence as a mother grew. I learned that there is no one-size-fits-all approach to motherhood. Each mother-child relationship is special and requires its own unique care. What worked for one family might not work for another, and that is okay. I embraced the journey of motherhood with all its imperfections, knowing that my love and dedication were the most valuable gifts I could give my baby boy.

Motherhood is an extraordinary journey, filled with a wide range of emotions and unique challenges. From the sleepless nights to the hormonal fluctuations, from the joys of breastfeeding to the overwhelming tiredness, it is a time of doubts, anxiety, and an abundance of unsolicited advice. This transformative phase has a name—it's called "matrescence."

In 1973, medical anthropologist Dana Raphael coined the term "matrescence" to describe the process of becoming a mother. It is akin to the concept of adolescence, and symbolizes the profound shift in a woman's life toward becoming a mother. It is important to distinguish matrescence from baby blues or postpartum depression, as it represents the multifaceted transformation of a woman as she embraces motherhood. Physically, hormonally, psychologically, and even spiritually, she undergoes a remarkable journey.

However, matrescence does not occur without challenges. Society often places an unspoken expectation that a new mother should feel nothing but pure joy after the arrival of her baby. This can create a lot of pressure and make it difficult for women to express a range of emotions, such as sadness, anxiety, or a loss of identity. Therefore, it is important to create a safe and understanding space where mothers can navigate the complexities of matrescence without facing judgment or criticism.

Let us celebrate the strength, resilience, and unconditional love that mothers possess. Instead of bombarding them with advice or suggestions, let us shower them with what they truly need—love and support. By normalizing the various emotions experienced during matrescence, we can create a nurturing environment in which mothers can explore their own unique journey of understanding their baby. Trusting their instincts and surrounding themselves with a supportive network can empower mothers to navigate the challenges of matrescence with self-compassion and grace.

Remember that you are not alone on this incredible journey. Embrace your own path, trust yourself, and seek out a community of support. Matrescence is a profound and beautiful transformation. As you embark on this new chapter, may you find strength, joy, and fulfillment in the remarkable role of motherhood.

The Baby Clash: A Journey of Transition from Couple to Parents

As Yamuna, entering into marriage with Mathan felt like opening a book with blank pages. Our families quickly brought our lives together, weaving our paths within just three short months. Here we were, living under the same roof, trying to navigate the unfamiliar terrain of our relationship, cautiously feeling our way through uncharted territory.

In the early days, our conversations were like tentative waves brushing against the shore. Our habits, our laughter, and our moments of silence slowly started to paint the picture of our newfound togetherness. Just as our bond was beginning to take shape, fate added a burst of color to the canvas—I discovered that I was pregnant.

The news bloomed within me like the first flower of spring; but it also brought a whirlwind of emotions. I felt like a young bird, eager yet unprepared to take flight. While my heart swelled with the joy of impending motherhood, deep down, I craved more time—time for Mathan and me to explore the uncharted waters of our marriage, time to grow as companions.

As the months went by, the reality of our baby's imminent arrival loomed large. Each passing day intensified the weight of impending motherhood, heightening my sense of unease. I questioned my readiness to shoulder the immense responsibility of nurturing a life and molding a tiny human into a responsible adult. Doubts about the strength of our relationship's foundation nagged at me, amplifying my concerns. The absence of a deep connection and a secure bond with my husband only added to my worries.

The birth of our baby brought a tidal wave of changes. Our once quiet home now echoed with the cries and coos of our newborn. As new parents, we found ourselves thrust into a whirlwind of sleepless nights and endless tasks. In the midst of countless diaper changes and feeding schedules, we felt like two strangers cohabiting, navigating this new territory separately, rather than as a united team.

The constant demands of parenthood left little space for us to revel in each other's company and savor moments of joy and companionship. I yearned for the days when our lives were not solely dictated by our little one's routines. I longed to build the deep connection that had eluded us in the whirlwind of our arranged marriage.

Yet, amid the challenges and uncertainties, we recognized that this was our reality—a tapestry woven with threads of love, duty, and shared responsibilities. We were a family, and we needed to find ways to fortify our bond and establish a rhythm that would harmonize our existence.

The road ahead was daunting, filled with uncertainty. But it was our journey—a path that we were destined to walk together. Our circumstances might have been unique, but the essence of our struggle was universal.

With each sleepless night and shared responsibility, we discovered more and more about each other—our strengths and weaknesses, fears and aspirations. Each day turned a new page in our story, offering opportunities to understand, compromise, and love.

The story of Yamuna and Mathan directs us to a real phenomenon called "the baby clash." The transition from being a couple to becoming parents is a seismic shift, one that can cause friction and create a chasm if not navigated sensitively. As per a 2021 study, one in three couples face a baby clash, with it being a common reason for separation.

There is a myriad of reasons for this, the most common ones being lack of communication, a sense of exclusion, misunderstandings, decreased intimacy, and a buildup of disagreements. Parenting, with its sleepless nights and relentless demands, is naturally stressful. Add to this the significant hormonal changes in a woman's body post-birth, and it's a veritable pressure cooker situation.

However, there are ways to alleviate this stress and bridge the gap. Open communication is the first step. Expressing your feelings honestly, without coating it with blame or criticism, can pave the way for understanding and empathy. Asking for help from family and friends, and outsourcing some tasks can free up your time for each other and help you reconnect.

There is a proverb that says, "it takes a village to raise a child"—and this proverb holds a profound truth. Distributing chores, finding time to rest and rejuvenate, and carving out pockets of "couple time" can help maintain a balance in your life after a baby. It is essential to understand that with the birth of a child, a new family is born—one that includes new roles for the mother and the father. These roles come with a learning curve and require time and patience to adapt.

The key is to remain patient, flexible, and open-minded. While the early months of parenthood can be challenging, they also offer an opportunity to strengthen the bond between couples, fostering a deeper sense of unity and shared purpose. It's a journey of growth and discovery, one that can be enriching and fulfilling if navigated with love, patience, and mutual respect.

Newborn Phase

The Power of Touch: Redefining Newborn Care in the 21st Century

In the realm of motherhood, I, Jenny, found myself standing on the cusp of a world, brimming with wonder. The arrival of my precious baby girl, a dream I held close, unfolded before me like a beautiful story.

But amid the soft wisps of her hair and the delicate touch of her tiny fingers, it seemed as though everyone around me had become self-appointed guardians of age-old maternal wisdom. My heart overflowed with affection, yet with each passing day, I found myself navigating through a storm of advice and admonitions.

"Don't kiss her like that!" "Don't hold her all the time!" The echoes of their words lingered in my ears. It was as though my natural instincts to nurture and protect were being restricted. But the one piece of advice that struck me deeply was the notion that I should let my baby cry, as a way to toughen her up and foster independence.

There she was, my heart residing outside my body, and yet, I was urged to let her cries go unanswered. They believed that detachment would prevent spoiling and encourage self-reliance. Some even claimed that letting the baby cry would strengthen their lungs and make them more resilient. These assertions left me torn. How could anyone understand that my deepest desire as a mother was to never let my newborn cry alone, and provide comfort and reassurance in their moments of distress?

No. My heart strongly disagreed to this notion. A baby enters this world seeking warmth, love, and security. They should feel the steady rhythm of the heart that nurtured them for nine months and know that they are cherished. Motherhood, to me, is not a rigid set of rules; it is an outpouring of unconditional love.

Long before my baby's arrival, I envisioned the profound bond that we would share. I dreamed of cradling my child, singing lullabies, sharing stories, and showering her with love. The directive to suppress these innate maternal instincts was disheartening and frustrating.

I firmly believe that my baby craves my unfiltered love and affection, and that cuddling is a means of expressing this profound emotion. It is not a path to spoiling a child, but rather a way of providing comfort and security. My deepest desire is for my child to grow up, knowing that they are deeply loved and that their mother will always be their safe haven.

The approach of letting the baby "cry it out" feels counterintuitive to me. It's like expecting a fledgling bird to fly without the initial guidance of its mother. How can I stand idly by, as a passive observer to my baby's distress? As a mother, every fiber of my being compels me to rush to my child, soothe their cries, and enfold them in a comforting embrace.

Moreover, I do not align with the belief that nursing and cradling my baby to sleep are detrimental practices. A wealth of studies suggests otherwise, asserting that these actions can actually cultivate healthy sleep patterns and foster a sense of security in babies. As a mother, my foremost concern is my baby's well-being. If that entails nursing and cradling them to sleep, I am more than willing to do so. As a new mother, my guiding principle is to drown out the clamor of unwarranted advice and listen to my maternal instincts.

In our society, a plethora of myths surround newborn care. These range from discouraging constant physical contact to promoting independence from day one. It is perplexing how society can expect a newborn, a being that has just entered the world, to be self-sufficient and manage their emotions independently.

This is the 21st century; a time when we understand the indelible imprint that early years have on one's soul. It's a time to cherish and uplift, to be present in the moment. The mental well-being we so fervently advocate must begin at the cradle.

Research asserts the undeniable power of touch. Numerous studies have unequivocally demonstrated that a baby cannot be spoiled by excess cuddling or holding. On the contrary, increased physical proximity can help the baby develop a sense of security and confidence. Additionally, physical closeness releases oxytocin and stimulates nerve fiber pathways, contributing to healthy brain development.

For preterm babies, the impact of gentle touch is even more profound. Regular, soft physical contact aids them in gaining strength and benefits their overall well-being.

Contrary to the myth, crying is a baby's unique language, their sole mode of expressing their needs. Ignoring their cries equates to overlooking their stress signals, pushing them into a state of greater stress. The remedy is simple: embrace them, assure them of their safety, and relieve their stress with a warm, comforting cuddle. This simple act unleashes the "love hormone," oxytocin, which plays a pivotal role in a child's overall development.

Harmonizing Traditions with Modern Parenthood: An Indian Perspective

Holding my baby boy tenderly, I crossed the doorway into the warm embrace of my parent's home, where my childhood had unfurled. The air, tinged with the aroma of mom's cooking, was a balm to my soul. My heart swelled with joy as my little one, just four months old, was about to experience the love and care that had nurtured me into the woman I am today. Yet, beneath the surface of my contentment, a concern was gnawing at me.

As I settled into the comforting nooks of the house, my family—my mother, grandmother, and siblings—bustled around us. Their laughter and the sound of clinking dishes formed the soundtrack of this new phase of my life. They were eager to lend a hand, watching over my baby while I snatched moments of rest. But there was this one matter where our thoughts collided—ragi milk.

Ragi milk, a traditional Indian drink made from finger millet, was the elixir of legends in my family. They firmly believed that it was the secret to their healthy children. They would narrate tales about how every infant in the family had thrived on it, myself included. The concept was so deeply ingrained in them that my decision to exclusively breastfeed my baby was met with shock and disapproval.

Every mealtime turned into a battlefield as I fought to resist the pressure of introducing ragi milk to my baby. I was determined to adhere to the World Health Organization's recommendations, which endorsed six months of exclusive breastfeeding. I tried to explain this to my family, but they dismissed my modern notions as whimsical.

"Your mother doesn't know anything," they'd murmur to my son, their voices laced with affection and a hint of condescension. "She herself drank ragi milk when she was a baby."

Their words cut through me, a painful reminder of the ongoing tug-of-war in our home. It was hurtful, especially when I was trying to do what I felt was best for my baby.

The situation was complex. I was extremely grateful for their help in attending to my little one. I could catch a few hours of sleep at night only because they took over some of the pressure. But the undercurrent of distrust, the fear that they might be feeding my baby ragi milk behind my back, kept me restless and on edge.

This predicament is not uncommon in Indian households. The older generation, having raised their children on a concoction of traditional practices, often find it difficult to adapt to new-age parenting norms. However, it is essential to remember that these actions stem from a place of love, albeit wrapped in an outdated cover of wisdom.

In the past, alternatives like ragi milk were introduced due to various reasons. The mother may have had difficulties in producing sufficient breast milk, or there may have been concerns about nutritional deficiencies. Thus, to ensure the baby was well-fed and received ample nutrition, practices like these were adopted.

Modern advancements in healthcare have since established the superiority of exclusive breastfeeding for the first six months of a child's life. A lactating mother's milk adapts to the changing nutritional needs of the baby. The newborn's digestive system, which is still in its development stage, can easily digest breast milk but would struggle with other forms of nutrition. Moreover, breastfeeding for the first six months significantly enhances the baby's immunity, making them better equipped to fight infections as they grow.

It is crucial for new mothers, particularly those in a similar predicament, to voice their concerns and fears clearly to their elders. Open conversations can help bridge the generational gap in understanding childcare practices. If need be, include them in postnatal medical appointments, where healthcare professionals can corroborate your views.

The journey of motherhood is filled with challenges and uncertainties. Navigating the uncharted waters of parenthood while keeping age-old family traditions at bay can seem like an uphill task. However, with patience, empathy, and open communication, it is possible to steer the ship toward the shores of a healthy and happy upbringing for your child. At the end of the day, everyone involved shares the same goal: the well-being of the baby. After all, it takes a village to raise a child.

Debunking the Indian Myths Around Pregnancy

In the tender symphony of the morning, as the sun kisses the horizon with hues of gold and amber, a village in the heartland of India stirs to life. In a quaint little house, an expecting mother caresses her belly, her eyes filled with dreams. The elders of the house have encircled her, and the air is rich with their whispers—whispers of ancient wisdom, age-old practices, and traditions passed down through generations like cherished heirlooms. Through a window, the aroma of earth and spices beckons her. The sanctity of this moment is almost palpable; it is as if time itself has slowed down to cradle her.

But wait, what's that we hear amid the whispers? "Don't eat that papaya!" "Apply this turmeric paste to have a fair child!" "Don't step out during an eclipse!" Ah, the web of myths that envelops Indian pregnancies!

Being an expectant mother in India is akin to being a vessel for not just a new life but also the entirety of the cultural heritage that you are expected to carry. In a land of astonishing diversity and deep-rooted traditions, pregnancy is more than a biological phenomenon; it is a tapestry woven with threads of myths, traditions, and an unyielding reverence for motherhood.

Some of these myths are so woven into the fabric of society that even modern, educated families find solace in adhering to them. Why? Perhaps, because there is a sense of belonging in tradition, a comfort in continuity.

But this is where the essence of our journey lies. Let us peek behind the veils of these myths, that are often tinged with a pinch of charm and a dash of mystique, and explore the truths that science and contemporary wisdom hold.

This is not just a catalog of myths and truths. It is, in its own way, a bridge between the past and the present; between the tender hopes of an expecting mother who, beneath the moonlit night, wishes upon a star, and the resolute voice of reason that whispers truths to the winds.

So, let's step into this wondrous garden of myths and truths, where each leaf tells a story and every bloom holds a secret. Together, let us seek, learn, and marvel at the tapestry that is pregnancy in India.

Myth: Consuming coconut water will help to ensure that the baby has a fair complexion

Under the shade of coconut trees, it is whispered among village folk that when a pregnant woman sips tender coconut water, it will bestow upon her child a fair complexion, akin to the pure, translucent water itself.

Truth:

Oh, how our imaginations soar! While coconut water is a treasure trove of electrolytes, minerals, and hydration, the color of your child's skin dances to the tunes of genetics. The genes inherited from both parents are the determinants of the child's skin color. So, while coconut water might nourish the body, it has no say in the complexion of your child's skin.

Myth: Eating papaya causes miscarriage

Wandering through the aromatic markets of India, you might hear a mother-in-law cautioning her pregnant daughter-in-law against consuming the luscious papaya, claiming that it's the harbinger of miscarriages.

Truth:

The truth is that unripe papaya does contain latex substances that might cause contractions. But ripe papayas are not only safe when consumed in moderation, they are also rich in antioxidants and vitamin C! They say wisdom ripens with age; let's say the same for papayas—as they ripen, they shed the myth and embrace the truth.

Myth: Wearing a safety pin protects against evil eyes

In bustling streets and serene hamlets, it is common to see pregnant women with a little safety pin attached inconspicuously to their clothes. This is believed to shield both mother and child from the piercing gaze of evil eyes.

Truth:

While the safety pin might not possess any mystical powers, its presence is a testament to the immense love and protective instincts that surround an expecting mother. There is no scientific evidence that a safety pin can fend off negative energies, but if it brings peace of mind and a sense of safety to the mother, perhaps that's a magic of its own.

Myth: The shape and fullness of the belly can indicate the baby's gender

In many a family gathering, you'll find relatives scrutinizing a pregnant woman's belly as though it is a crystal ball revealing mystical secrets. A high, round belly? It must be a girl! A low, spread-out one? Surely, a boy!

Truth:

Ah, the great belly oracle! But the reality is that the shape and fullness of a pregnant belly owe their form to factors like the mother's build and muscle tone, and the baby's position. As much as we love our family seers, science tells us that the belly's shape is not a gender radar. A baby's gender is determined by chromosomes, and the belly is simply the cozy abode where the baby grows.

Myth: Eating ghee will ensure a smooth delivery

The golden liquid that dances in pots across Indian kitchens, ghee, is often hailed as the secret potion for ensuring a smooth and quick delivery.

Truth:

While the thought of ghee acting as a lubricant does sound appealing, the birthing process is far more complex. Ghee is indeed a healthy fat and has its place in a balanced diet; but it does not possess any magical properties to ease labor. Smooth delivery is influenced by various factors including the baby's position, the mother's health, and sometimes sheer luck. Ghee might delight your taste buds, but let's leave easing of labor to medical science and the mother's strength.

Myth: Stepping out during an eclipse will cause birth defects in the child

It's as if time stands still during an eclipse in India, especially for pregnant women. It is believed that if a pregnant woman ventures out during an eclipse, the baby in her womb will develop birth defects. Hence, they are often advised to stay indoors, with some even adding an extra layer of protection by pinning leaves or amulets to their clothes.

Truth:

Eclipses are magnificent cosmic dances that do not sway the health of an unborn child in any way. Modern science confirms that an eclipse is a natural astronomical event that has no physical impact on pregnant women or their babies.

Myth: Sitting cross-legged will cause a cleft lip in the child

A common sight that you would see in Indian households is an anxious mother cautioning her pregnant daughter to avoid sitting cross-legged, lest her child be born with a cleft lip.

Truth:

Sitting cross-legged might be uncomfortable for some during pregnancy, but it has no bearing on whether the baby will have a cleft lip. Cleft lips arise from a combination of genetic and environmental factors. So, dear mothers-to-be, sit in whatever position you find comfortable and let the old wives' tales float away like whispers in the wind.

Myth: Consuming saffron will help you birth a fair-skinned baby

The golden strands of saffron, often considered worth their weight in gold, are believed by some to bequeath fair skin upon the unborn child.

Truth:

Saffron is a spice as rich in flavor as it is in history; but it does not have the power to paint the canvas of your child's skin. The tapestry of skin color is woven by genes, not by the spices in your kitchen. While adding saffron to the pregnant mother's milk might make for a delicious concoction, it does not hold the artist's brush to your baby's complexion.

Myth: Full moon means full term

There is an intriguing myth swirling around that full moons can trigger childbirth. Expectant parents often eagerly await the next full moon, hoping it's "the" night.

Truth:

Lunar cycles affecting childbirth is an age-old belief with a modern social media makeover. However, scientific studies have shown that there is no significant correlation between the phases of the moon and the likelihood of a pregnant woman going into labor. It is best to let nature take its course rather than consulting the lunar calendar!

Myth: Seeing something ugly or frightening can affect the baby's appearance

Some folks believe that if a pregnant woman sees something ugly or gets frightened, it might mark her unborn child.

Truth:

What your eyes behold does not have the power to sculpt your child's features. The development of a baby is a miraculous process governed by genetics and the prenatal environment. The symphony of life plays its own beautiful tune, irrespective of what crosses the expectant mother's path.

Myth: Craving salty foods means you're having a boy

Ah, the infamous craving compass! Many folks in India believe that if an expectant mother craves salty treats, it's a sign that she is carrying a baby boy.

Truth:

Cravings during pregnancy can be as unpredictable as a plot twist in a telenovela. Salty, sweet, or sour—cravings are typically driven by hormonal changes and nutritional needs, not by the baby's gender. Gender is determined by chromosomes, and no amount of salt can sway it!

Myth: A glowing mother will have a boy

It is believed that if a pregnant woman's face is glowing, she is going to have a boy; but if her beauty fades, expect a girl—they say a girl baby "steals her mother's beauty."

Truth:

Let's get real—pregnancy can make your skin go through all kinds of ups and downs due to hormonal changes. Glowing or not, it is no indicator of the baby's gender. And hey, every pregnant woman is beautiful in her own unique way.

Myth: Pregnant women should not attend funerals

There is a prevailing belief that attending funerals during pregnancy can attract negative energies that can affect the unborn child.

Truth:

While the notion of negative energies is more mystical than scientific, it is wise to consider the emotional toll that funerals can have on an expectant mother. The primary concern here should be the emotional well-being of the mother, as stress can have an impact on pregnancy.

Myth: A pregnant woman's face becoming round indicates that she is having a girl

Another facial fortune-telling! They say if a woman's face becomes rounder during pregnancy, she is carrying a girl.

Truth:

Facial changes, including swelling or rounding, are common during pregnancy due to fluid retention and hormonal shifts.

This is not a gender-revealing crystal ball, but a natural part of the pregnancy journey.

Myth: A pregnant woman should eat for two

This one's a classic, reborn in the age of Instagram food posts! Expectant mothers are encouraged to eat large portions because, after all, there is another human in there.

Truth:

While it is important for pregnant women to have a nutritious diet, "eating for two" is an exaggeration. An excessive caloric intake can lead to excessive weight gain and related health complications. It is more about eating smart rather than eating double.

Myth: Swinging your legs over the threshold will bring bad luck

In some parts of India, there's a peculiar myth that pregnant women should never swing their legs over the threshold while entering or leaving the house, as it is believed to bring bad luck.

Truth:

Crossing thresholds in any manner has no mystical power over luck. This myth probably originated as a cautionary tale to ensure that pregnant women are mindful of their movements to avoid tripping or falling. It's good to be cautious, but swinging your legs over a threshold does not have any control over luck or the well-being of the baby. So, let's set sail away from this one; it's just an old wives' tale that has no grounding in reality.

Myth: Evil eye will cause pregnancy complications

In many parts of India, it is believed that negative energies or the "evil eye" can cause complications during pregnancy. To ward this off, pregnant women are often adorned with black threads and charms.

Truth:

The concept of "evil eye" is deeply rooted in culture and folklore; but there is no scientific evidence supporting its existence or influence on pregnancy. It is important to focus on proven factors that contribute to a healthy pregnancy, like proper nutrition and regular check-ups.

Myth: You should not cut your hair during pregnancy

Scissors at the ready? Some believe that cutting hair during pregnancy can bring bad luck or harm to the baby.

Truth:

Snip away without worry! Cutting your hair has no effect on the health of the baby. This myth is based on cultural beliefs; but medically, there is no reason to avoid a trip to the salon.

Myth: Pregnant women should not look at fire

In certain regions, it is believed that looking at fire during pregnancy can affect the baby's eyesight.

Truth:

This one's a flickering myth without a spark of truth. Looking at fire does not have any effect on the unborn child's eyesight. The development of a baby's eyesight is influenced by genetics and the mother's overall health.

Myth: Crossing rivers during pregnancy can harm the baby

Some Indian communities believe that crossing rivers during pregnancy can cause harm to the unborn baby, as there are malevolent spirits in the water.

Truth:

As haunting as river spirits sound, there is no scientific basis for this myth. The health of a baby is influenced by various factors such as genetics, nutrition, and medical care, but surely not crossing bodies of water.

These myths woven into the very fabric of Indian culture have often guided generations of expectant mothers. However, with the beacon of science and reason, we have unraveled the threads and discerned myth from reality. Embracing these truths empowers us to make informed decisions and celebrate the profound journey of pregnancy with clarity and joy.

As we linger at the crossroads of tradition and modernity, we find new myths springing up like vibrant wildflowers in the age of social media. The next chapter will take you on a fresh adventure, as we decode the labyrinthine world of modern pregnancy myths that have taken root in the age of hashtags and viral posts. From avocadoes for brain development to exotic teas for painless labor, we will sift through the plethora of advice that fills our timelines.

The truths that we uncover may surprise you as much as the myths themselves.

Debunking the Modern Myths Around Pregnancy

With the clacking of keys and shimmering screens, we have stepped into the pulsating heart of the digital age. Here, in this cornucopia of information, where whispers become roars with a single click, we find a new landscape of myths blooming amid tweets and hashtags.

Picture this: A woman finds out that she is pregnant. She is elated, nervous, and keen to know all there is to know about this journey she is about to embark on. She reaches for her smartphone, and as she scrolls through her feed, she is inundated with a cascade of posts, articles, and unsolicited advice. There is a celebrity endorsing a pregnancy tea, a blogger swearing by a particular yoga pose, and endless forums discussing every imaginable pregnancy quirk. It's a deluge and she's barely got an umbrella!

Let's pause and ask ourselves: "What is the real flavor of the myths marinating in the social media sauce?" They're international, borderless, and often fancily dressed. They dance on our screens with the allure of newness and the promise of insider knowledge. Are avocados the magical fruit for brain development? Is there an app that can sing lullabies to your unborn child? Can your baby taste the garlic bread you ate for dinner?

In this whirlwind chapter, we shall don our digital explorer hats and delve into these vibrant, often amusing, but sometimes worrying modern myths about pregnancy.

Myth: Using a fetal doppler at home is a great way to bond with your baby

Social media feeds are replete with images of happy parents-to-be using at-home fetal dopplers to listen to their baby's heartbeat. It's touted as a bonding experience.

Truth:

Hold on to your dopplers, folks! Frequent use of fetal dopplers at home isn't recommended by healthcare professionals. These devices can give inaccurate readings, causing unnecessary panic or false reassurance. It is best to leave the monitoring of your baby's heartbeat to your healthcare provider during scheduled prenatal visits.

Myth: Applying coconut oil on the belly will help prevent stretch marks

Numerous posts and articles claim that applying coconut oil religiously on the belly will help prevent the occurrence of stretch marks during pregnancy.

Truth:

While coconut oil can keep the skin moisturized, it is not a magic elixir for preventing stretch marks. Stretch marks are influenced by factors such as genetics, the rate of weight gain, and skin elasticity. It is okay to use coconut oil for moisturization, but it is essential to have realistic expectations.

Myth: Wearing a rose quartz crystal ensures a calm pregnancy

There is a buzz around wearing rose quartz crystal, claiming that it harmonizes emotions and guarantees a calm and serene pregnancy.

Truth:

Wearing rose quartz or any crystal can be aesthetically pleasing and even serve as a comforting ritual for some; but there is no scientific evidence to support the notion that crystals have any tangible effect on a pregnant woman's emotional state. A calm and serene state of mind can be achieved through a combination of factors including support, self-care, and sometimes professional help.

Myth: Eating spicy food will induce labor

Posts on social media often claim that eating spicy food is a surefire way to induce labor.

Truth:

There is no scientific backing to the claim that spicy food can induce labor. While some women might experience contractions due to the gastrointestinal distress caused by spicy foods, this shouldn't be confused with the onset of labor. It is best to not rely on spicy foods for labor induction.

Myth: Drinking raspberry leaf tea will make labor shorter

You might come across several enthusiastic posts advocating the consumption of raspberry leaf tea when you go into labor, claiming that it makes labor significantly short and less painful.

Truth:

Although raspberry leaf tea has been associated with toning the uterus, there is no strong scientific evidence that supports the claims of it making labor shorter or less painful. It is essential to consult with your healthcare provider before including any herbal tea in your diet during pregnancy.

Myth: Good hip size or small babies make for an easier birth

It is popularly believed that a pregnant woman's good hip size or a baby's small built can lead to an easier birth.

Truth:

Contrary to this belief, there is no scientific evidence to support the notion that good hip size or small baby can lead to an easier birth. The ease or difficulty of labor depends on various factors such as the baby's position, the mother's contractions, the flexibility of her pelvic ligaments, and her overall health.

Myth: You can drink a glass or two of wine while pregnant

In today's world, it is believed that pregnant women can drink a glass or two of wine, and that it will not harm them or their baby.

Truth:

It is crucial to understand that consuming alcohol during pregnancy and childbirth is strongly discouraged. Even small amounts of alcohol can pose serious risks to the developing fetus, leading to a range of potential complications and lifelong consequences. To prioritize the health and well-being of the baby, it is recommended to abstain from alcohol entirely during pregnancy and childbirth.

Myth: Eating avocado will boost your baby's brain development

Social media is brimming with posts about the miracle of avocados, touting them as the ultimate brain-boosting food for your unborn baby.

Truth:

While avocados are undeniably nutritious and contain healthy fats and folate, attributing brain-boosting superpowers specifically to them is exaggeration. A balanced diet with a variety of fruits and vegetables, including avocados, can contribute to the overall health of both the mother and the baby.

Myth: Eating chocolate will make your baby happier

Some posts claim that consuming chocolate while pregnant will result in a happier baby.

Truth:

Eating chocolate in moderation can be a delightful indulgence for expecting mothers, but it does not directly make your baby happier. It is important to maintain a balanced diet and ensure a healthy lifestyle for the well-being of both the mother and the baby.

Myth: Facial recognition apps can almost predict your baby's face

Social media is buzzing with apps that claim to predict how your baby will look by analyzing the parents' pictures.

Truth:

While this may be a fun activity for expectant parents, these apps are not based on science and are simply meant for entertainment purposes. The baby's appearance is determined by complex genetic factors and cannot be accurately predicted by an app.

Whispers of the Heart: Pregnancy Affirmations

As you traverse the miraculous journey of motherhood, it is important to remember that both your mind and your body are undergoing significant transformations. It's a time of creation, nurturing, and blooming. Yet, it can also be a time of uncertainties, questions, and doubts. But, dear reader, always remember that these highs and lows are both different strokes of the same beautiful painting called pregnancy. This section of the book is dedicated to you—the radiant expectant mothers, who are the real-life superheroes. We present you with a series of affirmations—soothing words that will serve as your beacons, gently guiding you through the intricate labyrinth of pregnancy. As you embrace each of these affirmations, allow them to seep into your being, fortify your spirit, and nourish your journey to motherhood.

"I am capable, I am resilient."

Motherhood is a testament to your incredible strength and resilience. There will be challenging days, but always remember that you are capable of withstanding these obstacles. Your strength comes not just from your physical being, but also from the depth of your emotions, the courage of your spirit, and the resilience that each moment of motherhood imbues in you.

"My body is performing a miracle."

There is no greater wonder than the one your body is currently undertaking. It is essential to respect, appreciate, and love your body for this beautiful process. Each stretch mark that forms on your belly is a sign of your body's adaptability, and every pound that you gain is a symbol of the life you are nurturing.

"I trust in my body's wisdom."

Your body has innate wisdom that guides it through the process of creating and nurturing life. It knows when to rest, when to surge with energy, and when to crave particular nutrients. Trusting your body is equal to trusting nature's grand design of motherhood.

"I am connected with my baby."

Even before you hold your baby in your arms, you are intricately connected with this new life. This bond is not just physical, but emotional and spiritual too. Every heartbeat and every movement strengthens this connection.

"I embrace the changes with love and patience."

Pregnancy is a symphony of change—physical, emotional, and spiritual. Embrace each change with love, for these changes are molding you into a mother. Practice patience with yourself and your body as you navigate these shifts. The journey to motherhood is not a race, but a transformative path to be experienced and treasured.

"I am surrounded by love and support."

Sometimes, it may feel like you are walking this path alone; but remember that there is an aura of love and support that envelops you. From your family and friends to fellow moms-to-be, you are part of a tapestry of love that will buoy you through this journey.

"My instincts are my guiding stars."

As an expecting mother, you will receive advice from various quarters. While they may be well-intentioned, not all advice may resonate with you. Trust your maternal instincts; they are the whispers of your heart that will seldom lead you astray. Your inner voice is your most authentic guide.

"I am a source of life, beauty, and grace."

Embrace the fact that as a life-bearer, you are a wellspring of beauty and grace. Your glow is not just external but emanates from within as you carry the miracle of life. Bask in this grace and allow it to radiate outward, touching all those around you.

"I honor my journey with compassion for myself."

Be kind and gentle to yourself. Your pregnancy journey is unique, and comparing it with that of others will only create unnecessary pressure. Honor your personal voyage by giving yourself grace, understanding, and most importantly, compassion in every step.

"I am preparing to welcome immeasurable love into my life."

You are on the threshold of experiencing a love that knows no bounds. The love between a mother and her child is an endless ocean, vast and deep. As you prepare for this momentous milestone, know that your heart and life are about to be enriched in ways you never thought possible.

Reflections of Motherhood—A Journal

As you stand on the precipice of motherhood, a symphony of emotions swirls within you—elation, dreams, tenderness, and perhaps a whisper of trepidation. This haven within the pages of our book is your soft, warm embrace; a serene sanctuary that holds your hand as you weave the threads of your being with the new soul blossoming inside you.

In this sanctuary, we shall waltz through the hallowed grounds of journaling—a journey that invites your heart to sail across the oceans of your emotions, with questions as your compass. Our purpose is to awaken the depths of your soul, clear the mists of your heart, and kindle a luminescence within you. With each pen stroke, feel the alchemy of your words transform your path into an odyssey of love.

What does becoming a mother mean to me?

Peel back the layers of your soul. What songs does your heart sing at the thought of motherhood? Paint your emotions on this canvas with abandon.

How am I feeling about my body's changes?

Your body is a sacred tapestry being woven anew. Celebrate the marvels it is unfolding; it is a living testament to life's greatest miracle.

What strengths am I bringing into motherhood?

Inside you is a boundless reservoir of gifts and treasures. What do you carry into this sacred mantle of motherhood?

How can I best nurture myself during pregnancy?

Nourishing your being is an act of boundless love. How will you cradle your essence with tenderness during this time?

What do I hope for my child?

What are the dreams that take flight on your heart's wings for your cherished one? Let your hopes bloom through your words.

How do I imagine my relationship with my baby?

Picture the tapestry of love and connection that you and your little one will weave together. What colors, textures, and patterns does it bear?

What fears or anxieties do I need to address?

Let's gather the shadows that may cloud your path, and with grace, release them into the ether. Pen them down and allow them to dissolve.

What does a positive birthing experience look like for me?

You have the power to shape your birth story. What chapters of triumph, joy, and strength will it behold?

How am I preparing myself mentally and emotionally for motherhood?

Motherhood is an expedition of the soul. How are you charting the landscapes of your inner world for this journey?

What support do I need and who can provide it?

Behind you stands an invisible tapestry of love and support. Who do you trust to be the guardians of your sanctuary?

This sacred alcove is yours to cultivate and nourish. Within these questions lies an invitation for your heart to unfurl its petals.

As we turn the final page of this book, let's pause for a moment and cherish the beautiful journey you're on. You've taken bold steps, asked important questions, and reflected deeply. But let's not close the book here.

There's more in store!

I've got a special companion for you—*'Blooming Belly: A pregnancy journal"*.

Your voice, your story, and your heart—this journal is a canvas waiting for you.

Scan the QR code below to grab your very own "Blooming Belly: A pregnancy journal". Make it your confidant, your daily check-in, where you record your laughter and tears through this roller coaster of wonders.

[QR CODE]

www.ingramcontent.com/pod-product-compliance
Lightning Source LLC
LaVergne TN
LVHW091047150826
845673LV00002B/495

9798890669490